V VETERINARY

M MEDICAL

S SCHOOL

A° ADMISSION

R REQUIREMENTS

in the

United States

and Canada

WITHDRAWN

St. Louis Community College
at Meramec
Library

WITHDRAWN

VETERINARY MEDICAL SCHOOL ADMISSION REQUIREMENTS

in the
United States and Canada

2000 Edition for 2001 Matriculation

Association of American
Veterinary Medical Colleges

PURDUE UNIVERSITY PRESS   WEST LAFAYETTE, INDIANA

Copyright ©2000 by the Association of American Veterinary
Medical Colleges. All rights reserved.

∞™ The paper used in this book meets the minimum requirements
of American National Standard for Information Sciences —
Permanence of Paper for Printed Library Materials, ANSI Z39.48-1992.

Cover photo: Clinical experience is a vital and often enjoyable part of veterinary medical education.
Photo courtesy Mississippi State University College of Veterinary Medicine.

Printed in the United States of America

ISBN 1-55753-219-2
ISSN 1089-6465

Contents

Foreword

The opportunities and options for veterinarians are more varied than ever. Today's veterinary student can choose to train for a career in environmental problem-solving, local community health, food resource management, zoo animal care, space and marine biology, or wildlife preservation in addition to the more traditional small- or large-animal practice.

The choices begin with selecting and applying to the right veterinary medical schools. An uninformed decision could lead to costly mistakes, or even academic failure. Students, parents, mentors, and counselors need help to make sure that such important decisions are based on sound knowledge, and *Veterinary Medical School Admission Requirements (VMSAR)* is an invaluable source for this essential information.

This 16th edition provides current information for all thirty-one veterinary medical schools in the United States and Canada. The entry for each school includes information on the admissions office contact, prerequisite courses, application deadlines, standardized test requirements, residency implications, timetables, cost of education, and other admission policies and procedures. This book also includes information on special programs, statistical data on the national applicant pool, and minority student opportunities. A valuable new feature, "Financing Your Veterinary Medical Education," was provided by Deb Burdick, assistant director at Iowa State University's Office of Student Financial Aid.

VMSAR is compiled annually under the auspices of the Association of American Veterinary Medical Colleges (AAVMC). The AAVMC welcomes suggestions for future editions; they may be directed to Denise A. Ottinger, Director of Student Services, 1240 Lynn Hall, School of Veterinary Medicine, Purdue University, West Lafayette, Indiana 47907-1240.

My thanks to each of the veterinary medical schools for their assistance in making this book possible each year.

Denise A. Ottinger, Editor
School of Veterinary Medicine at Purdue University

Abbreviations

AAVMC	Association of American Veterinary Medical Colleges
AVMA	American Veterinary Medical Association
BA/BS	Bachelor of Arts or Bachelor of Science degrees
CVMA	Canadian Veterinary Medical Association
DVM/VMD	Doctor of Veterinary Medicine degree
GRE	Graduate Record Examination
MCAT	Medical College Admission Test
MPH	Master of Public Health
MPVM	Master of Preventive Veterinary Medicine degree
MS	Master of Science degree
PhD	Doctor of Philosophy degree
SREB	Southern Regional Education Board
TOEFL	Test of English as a Foreign Language
VCAT	Veterinary College Admission Test
VMCAS	Veterinary Medical College Application Service
VMD/DVM	Veterinary Medical Doctor degree
VMSAR	Veterinary Medical School Admission Requirements
WICHE	Western Interstate Commission for Higher Education

Veterinary Medicine: Choices and Challenges

Considered from the perspective of comparative medicine, veterinarians help animals and people live longer, healthier lives. They serve society by preventing and treating animal disease, improving the quality of the environment, ensuring the safety of food, controlling diseases transmitted from animals, and advancing medical knowledge. The Doctor of Veterinary Medicine degree can lead to diverse career opportunities and different lifestyles from a solo mixed-animal practice in a rural area to a teaching or research position at an urban university, medical center, or industrial laboratory. The majority of veterinarians in the United States are in private practice, although significant numbers are involved in preventive medicine, regulatory veterinary medicine, military veterinary medicine, laboratory animal medicine, research and development in industry, and teaching and research in a variety of basic science and clinical disciplines.

License to Practice

The DVM (or VMD) degree is awarded after 4 years of successful study at an accredited college of veterinary medicine. Graduate veterinarians are eligible to apply for a license to practice. Licensing is controlled by states and provinces, each of which has rules and procedures for legal practice within its own jurisdiction. All require satisfactory completion of the national board examination, and most have other requirements, including additional tests and interviews.

Specialization

Graduate veterinarians may choose to become specialists in a clinical area or to work with particular species. The first step on the path toward specialization is usually an internship.

Internship

Internships are 1-year programs in either small- or large-animal medicine and surgery. The most prestigious internship programs are at veterinary medical colleges or at very large private veterinary hospitals with board-certified veterinarians on staff. Since internships are usually at large referral centers, interns are exposed to a larger number of challenging cases than they would be likely to see in a smaller private practice.

Veterinary students in their senior year and veterinary graduates apply for internships through a matching program. Internship applicants and training hospitals rank each other in order of preference, and a computerized system matches each applicant with the highest-ranking teaching hospital that ranked the applicant. Academic performance in the veterinary professional curriculum, as well as recommendations from veterinary school faculty, is considered in the ranking of internship applicants.

Most veterinary interns in the United States receive a nominal salary, and their educational debts, if any, may be postponed in some governmentally subsidized loan programs. Veterinarians can often command a higher starting salary in private practice after completion of an internship. Also, an internship is the next step, after receiving the DVM degree, toward residency and board certification.

Residency Training

Veterinarians who complete internships or who have 2 years of private-practice experience are eligible to apply for residency programs. Residency training is more specialized than an internship. Currently, residency training is available in internal medicine, surgery, cardiology, dermatology, ophthalmology, exotic small animal medicine, pathology, neurology, radiology, anesthesiology, and oncology. The programs take 2 to 3 years to complete, depending on the nature of the specialty. Successful completion of a residency is required for certification by any of the veterinary medical specialty boards. Some residencies combine research and graduate study to lead to a master's degree.

Board Certification

Veterinary board certification and diplomate status are available for 20 specialties: anesthesiology, animal behavior, clinical pharmacology, dentistry, dermatology, emergency and critical care, internal medicine, laboratory animal medicine, microbiology, nutrition, ophthalmology, pathology, poultry medicine, private practice, preventive medicine, radiology, surgery, theriogenology (reproduction), toxicology, and zoological medicine.

Private and Public Practice

A significant percentage of veterinary graduates are engaged in private practice, either as an owner of a solo practice or, more likely, as a partner or associate in a group practice. Increasingly, veterinarians work together as a team, which allows a wider range of services to be provided.

Small-animal veterinarians focus their efforts primarily on dogs and cats but are seeing a growing number of pet birds and exotic animals such as reptiles.

Veterinarians specializing in large animals often place their emphasis on horses, cattle, or pigs, and work both on a farm-call and an in-clinic basis. A mixed-animal veterinarian works with all types of animals.

Some veterinarians obtain further specialization in such areas as diseases or disorders of the eyes of cats or reproduction difficulties in cattle.

Public practice provides a variety of opportunities at the national, state, county, or city levels. Opportunities in food safety, public health, the military, animal disease control, research, and the care and maintenance of wildlife abound.

Industry

Veterinarians have many opportunities available to them in private industry, particularly in the fields of nutrition and pharmaceuticals. Assisting in the development of new products in the animal industry, conducting research for pharmaceutical companies, diagnosing disease and drug effects as pathologists, or safeguarding the health of laboratory animal colonies are all interesting career possibilities. Some veterinarians may be employed by zoos and aquariums and may act as consultants to wildlife preservation groups, game farms, or fisheries.

New or Unusual Career Opportunities

By the very nature of the many species of animals involved and the wide variety of clientele served, the opportunities available to today's veterinarian are abundant. The role of the veterinarian in society has changed and evolved over time, so that they are now specially qualified to take part in many problems related to the environment, local community health, food resource management, zoo animal care, space and marine biology, and wildlife preservation.

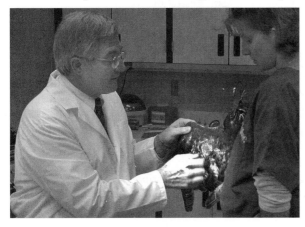

Examining an injured red-tailed hawk is all in a day's work at the Southeastern Raptor Rehabilitation Center at Auburn University's College of Veterinary Medicine. Photo courtesy of Auburn University College of Veterinary Medicine.

3

Alphabetical Listing of Veterinary Schools

United States

Auburn University	Auburn University, Alabama
California, University of	Davis, California
Colorado State University	Fort Collins, Colorado
Cornell University	Ithaca, New York
Florida, University of	Gainesville, Florida
Georgia, University of	Athens, Georgia
Illinois, University of	Urbana, Illinois
Iowa State University	Ames, Iowa
Kansas State University	Manhattan, Kansas
Louisiana State University	Baton Rouge, Louisiana
Michigan State University	East Lansing, Michigan
Minnesota, University of	St. Paul, Minnesota
Mississippi State University	Mississippi State, Mississippi
Missouri, University of	Columbia, Missouri
North Carolina State University	Raleigh, North Carolina
Ohio State University	Columbus, Ohio
Oklahoma State University	Stillwater, Oklahoma
Oregon State University	Corvallis, Oregon
Pennsylvania, University of	Philadelphia, Pennsylvania
Purdue University	West Lafayette, Indiana
Tennessee, University of	Knoxville, Tennessee
Texas A & M University	College Station, Texas
Tufts University	North Grafton, Massachusetts
Tuskegee University	Tuskegee, Alabama
Virginia Polytechnic Institute and State University (Virginia-Maryland Regional)	Blacksburg, Virginia
Washington State University	Pullman, Washington
Wisconsin, University of	Madison, Wisconsin

Canada

Guelph, University of	Guelph, Ontario
Montréal, Université de	Montréal, Québec
Prince Edward Island, University of	Charlottetown, Prince Edward Island
Saskatchewan, University of	Saskatoon, Saskatchewan

Geographical Listing of Veterinary Schools and Directory of Admissions Offices

United States

Alabama

Office for Academic Affairs
College of Veterinary Medicine
217 Goodwin Student Center
Auburn University
Auburn University AL 36849-5536

College of Veterinary Medicine,
    Nursing, and Allied Health
Tuskegee University
Tuskegee AL 36088

California

Office of the Dean-Student Programs
School of Veterinary Medicine
One Shields Avenue
Surge IV
University of California
Davis CA 95616

Colorado

Office of the Dean
College of Veterinary Medicine and
    Biomedical Sciences
Colorado State University
Fort Collins CO 80523-1601

Florida

Office for Students and Instruction
College of Veterinary Medicine
P.O. Box 100125
University of Florida
Gainesville FL 32610-0125

Georgia

Office for Academic Affairs
College of Veterinary Medicine
The University of Georgia
Athens GA 30602-7372

Illinois

Office of Academic and Student
    Affairs
College of Veterinary Medicine
University of Illinois at Urbana-
    Champaign
2271G Veterinary Medicine Basic
    Sciences Bldg.
2001 South Lincoln Avenue
Urbana IL 61802

Indiana

Student Services Office
School of Veterinary Medicine
1240 Lynn Hall
Purdue University
West Lafayette IN 47907-1240

Iowa

Office of Admissions
Room 100 Alumni Hall
Iowa State University
Ames IA 50011-2011

Kansas
Office of Admissions
College of Veterinary Medicine
101 Trotter Hall
1700 Denison Avenue
Kansas State University
Manhattan KS 66506-5601

Louisiana
Office of Veterinary Student Affairs
School of Veterinary Medicine
Louisiana State University
Baton Rouge LA 70803

Massachusetts
Office of Admissions
School of Veterinary Medicine
200 Westboro Road
Tufts University
North Grafton MA 01536

Michigan
Office of Admissions
College of Veterinary Medicine
A-126 East Fee Hall
Michigan State University
East Lansing MI 48824-1316

Minnesota
Office of Student Affairs and
  Admissions
College of Veterinary Medicine
460 Veterinary Teaching Hospital
1365 Gortner Avenue
University of Minnesota
St. Paul MN 55108

Mississippi
Admissions Coordinator
College of Veterinary Medicine
P.O. Box 9825
Mississippi State University
Mississippi State MS 39762

Missouri
Office of Academic Affairs
College of Veterinary Medicine
W203 Veterinary Medicine Building
University of Missouri-Columbia
Columbia MO 65211

New York
Office of DVM Admissions
College of Veterinary Medicine
S2-009 Schurman Hall
Cornell University
Ithaca NY 14853-6401

North Carolina
Student Services Office
College of Veterinary Medicine
4700 Hillsborough Street
North Carolina State University
Raleigh NC 27606

Ohio
Chairperson, Admissions Committee
College of Veterinary Medicine
0004 Veterinary Hospital
601 Tharp Street
The Ohio State University
Columbus OH 43210-1089

Oklahoma
Admissions Office
College of Veterinary Medicine
Oklahoma State University
Stillwater OK 74078-2003

Oregon
Office of the Dean
College of Veterinary Medicine
Oregon State University
200 Magruder Hall
Corvallis OR 97331-4801

Pennsylvania
Admissions Office
School of Veterinary Medicine
3800 Spruce Street
University of Pennsylvania
Philadelphia PA 19104-6044

Tennessee
Office of the Associate Dean
College of Veterinary Medicine
P.O. Box 1071
University of Tennessee
Knoxville TN 37901-1071

Texas
Office of the Dean
College of Veterinary Medicine
Texas A & M University
College Station TX 77843-4461

Virginia
Admissions Coordinator
Virginia-Maryland Regional College
  of Veterinary Medicine
Virginia Polytechnic Institute and
  State University
Blacksburg VA 24061

Washington
Office of Student Services
College of Veterinary Medicine
Washington State University
Pullman WA 99164-7012

Wisconsin
Office of Academic Affairs
School of Veterinary Medicine
2015 Linden Drive West
University of Wisconsin-Madison
Madison WI 53706-1102

Canada

Montréal
Service des Admissions
Université de Montréal
C.P. 6205
Succursale Centre-Ville
Montréal Québec H3C 3T5

Ontario
Admissions Services
University Centre, Level 3
University of Guelph
Guelph Ontario N1G 2W1

Prince Edward Island
Registrar's Office
Atlantic Veterinary College
University of Prince Edward Island
550 University Avenue
Charlottetown PEI C1A 4P3

Saskatchewan
Admissions Office
Western College of Veterinary
    Medicine
University of Saskatchewan
52 Campus Drive
Saskatoon Saskatchewan S7N 5B4

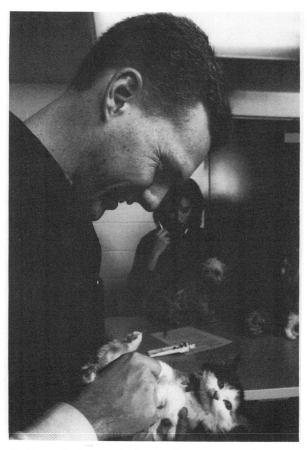

Providing medical care to animals at area Humane Societies allows veterinary students at Oklahoma State University hands-on training while also benefiting the animals. Photo courtesy Oklahoma State University College of Veterinary Medicine.

LISTING OF SCHOOLS ACCEPTING NONRESIDENT/NONCONTRACT APPLICATIONS

United States	Number of Positions Available
Auburn University	10 positions; U.S. citizens only.
University of California	Limited number of positions.
Colorado State University	10-20 positions; international applicants considered.
Cornell University	20-26 positions available; international applicants considered.
University of Florida	Not more than 15% of entering class.
University of Georgia	Up to 10 positions.
University of Illinois	20 positions.
Iowa State University	10-25 positions available, plus unfilled contract positions; international applicants considered.
Kansas State University	15-20% of class, plus unfilled contract positions; international applicants considered.
Louisiana State University	Not more than 10% of entering class.
Michigan State University	Not more than 20-25% of entering class; international applicants considered.
University of Minnesota	Not more than 20% of entering class.
Mississippi State University	19 positions.
University of Missouri	10 positions.
North Carolina State University	12 positions.
Ohio State University	Up to 30 positions.
Oklahoma State University	Up to 14 positions.

Oregon State University	Up to 8 positions.
University of Pennsylvania	45-50 positions; international applicants considered.
Purdue University	20 positions available; international applicants considered.
University of Tennessee	Limited number of positions.
Texas A & M University	Up to 8 positions.
Tufts University	35-40 positions.
Tuskegee University	Up to 10 positions; international applicants considered.
Virginia-Maryland Regional College of Veterinary Medicine	Up to 10 positions.
Washington State University	Limited number of positions.
University of Wisconsin	10-20 positions.

Canada

University of Prince Edward Island	19 positions for international applicants.

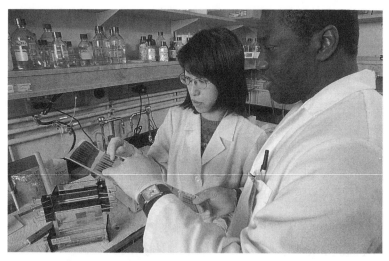

Many veterinary medical students choose a career in research rather than a clinical practice.
Photo by Vincent P. Walter, courtesy Office of Publications, Purdue University.

LISTING OF CONTRACTING STATES AND PROVINCES

All Canadian provinces and 20 states in the United States that do not have a veterinary school contract with one or more schools to provide access to veterinary medical education for their residents. The state or province, working through the contracting agency, usually agrees to pay a fee to help cover the cost of education for a certain number of places in each entering class. Residents from the contract states then compete with each other for those positions.

Some states contract with more than one school. For example, Arkansas contracts with 5 veterinary schools, and North Dakota has contracts with 6 schools. Connecticut, Rhode Island, Vermont, and the District of Columbia presently have no contracts, so all candidates from these places apply as nonresidents to veterinary schools of their choice.

The educational agreements between contracting agencies and veterinary schools differ. Under some contract arrangements, students pay in-state tuition; in others, they pay nonresident tuition. Some contract states require students to repay all or part of the subsidy that the state provided; others require veterinary graduates to return to practice in the state for a period of time. Applicants should be aware of their obligation to the state before agreeing to participate in a contract program.

Following is a list of states and provinces that have educational agreements with schools of veterinary medicine.

UNITED STATES

Alaska
Contracts through WICHE* with University of California, Colorado State University, Oregon State University, and Washington State University.

Arizona
Contracts through WICHE* with University of California, Colorado State University, Oregon State University, and Washington State University.

Arkansas
Contracts in past with Tuskegee University, Louisiana State University, Mississippi State University, University of Missouri, and Oklahoma State University. Contracts not all completed at time of printing; may be some changes.

Delaware
Contracts with Virginia-Maryland Regional College.

* WICHE = Western Interstate Commission for Higher Education (offices in Boulder, Colorado)

Georgia
Contracts with Tuskegee University, in addition to having a school in the state.

Hawaii
Contracts through WICHE* with University of California, Colorado State University, Oregon State University, and Washington State University.

Idaho
Contracts with Washington State University.

Kentucky
Contracts with Auburn University and Tuskegee University.

Maine
Contracts with Tufts University.

Montana
Contracts through WICHE* with University of California, Colorado State University, Oregon State University, and Washington State University.

Nebraska
Contracts with Kansas State University.

Nevada
Contracts through WICHE* with University of California, Colorado State University, Oregon State University, and Washington State University; and also with Ohio State University.

New Hampshire
Contracts with Cornell University and Tufts University.

New Jersey
Contracts with Cornell University, University of Illinois, Iowa State University, University of Pennsylvania, Oklahoma State University, Tufts University, and Tuskegee University.

New Mexico
Contracts through WICHE* with University of California, Colorado State University, Oregon State University, and Washington State University.

North Dakota
Reciprocity with University of Minnesota. Contracts with Iowa State University. Contracts through WICHE* with University of California, Colorado State University, Oregon State University, and Washington State University.

* WICHE = Western Interstate Commission for Higher Education (offices in Boulder, Colorado)

Puerto Rico
Contracts with Cornell University and Tuskegee University. Cooperative agreement with University of Wisconsin.

South Carolina
Contracts with University of Georgia and Tuskegee University.

South Dakota
Reciprocity with University of Minnesota. Contracts with Iowa State University.

Utah
Contracts through WICHE* with University of California, Colorado State University, Oregon State University, and Washington State University.

West Virginia
Contracts with University of Georgia, Ohio State University, and Tuskegee University.

Wyoming
Contracts through WICHE* with the University of California, Colorado State University, Oregon State University, and Washington State University.

CANADA

Alberta
Contracts with University of Saskatchewan.

British Columbia
Contracts with University of Saskatchewan.

Manitoba
Reciprocity with University of Minnesota. Contracts with University of Saskatchewan.

New Brunswick
Contracts with Atlantic Veterinary College at the University of Prince Edward Island.

Newfoundland
Contracts with Atlantic Veterinary College at the University of Prince Edward Island.

Northwest Territories
Contracts with University of Saskatchewan.

Nova Scotia
Contracts with Atlantic Veterinary College at the University of Prince Edward Island.

Yukon Territory
Contracts with University of Saskatchewan.

* WICHE = Western Interstate Commission for Higher Education (offices in Boulder, Colorado)

Programs for Multicultural or Disadvantaged Students

The Association of American Veterinary Medical Colleges affirms the value of diversity within the veterinary medical profession. The membership is committed to incorporating that belief into their actions by advocating the recruitment and retention of underrepresented persons as students and faculty and ultimately fostering their success in the profession of veterinary medicine. The Association believes that through these actions society and the profession will be well served.

Many schools have programs designed to facilitate entry into, and retention by, veterinary programs nationwide. These programs are directed at several levels, from high-school students to the student who has already been accepted by a veterinary college. Most of these programs will accept students from every state, regardless of the school(s) to which an individual might eventually apply or attend.

Following is an alphabetical list of schools by state and a short explanation of their programs:

Auburn University College of Veterinary Medicine
Program: Summer Laboratory Experiences for High School Students

Description: students who have demonstrated an interest in the biological or health sciences spend 8 weeks working in the laboratory of a senior research scientist. Whenever possible, students will design and conduct an experiment and present the results to students and faculty during an exit seminar. Orientation sessions provide the student with the basics of laboratory safety and an introduction to sterile technique. An enrichment program provides information on career-related opportunities and cultural programs.

Eligibility: minority high-school students who have completed the junior or senior year with strong grades in science and recommendations from their teachers are considered.

Contact: Coordinator of Recruiting, College of Veterinary Medicine, Auburn University AL 36849-5519; telephone: (334) 844-2685; fax: (334) 844-2723.

Sponsorship: National Institutes of Health, National Center for Research Resources.

University of California

Program: Summer Enrichment Program

Description: a 6-week summer residential program. The purpose of this program is to increase the academic preparedness of disadvantaged students through science-based learning skills development, clinical education, individual advising, and student development.

Eligibility: junior, senior, or postbaccalaureate student. Educationally and/or economically disadvantaged. Must have a cumulative undergraduate and required science GPA of 2.50 and demonstrated interest in veterinary medicine.

Program dates: July–August.

Contact: Office of the Dean, School of Veterinary Medicine, University of California, One Shields Avenue, Davis CA 95616; telephone: (530) 752-1383.

Sponsorship: School of Veterinary Medicine, University of California-Davis.

Colorado State University

Program: Vet Start

Description: a 7-year undergraduate and professional program for students who come to Colorado State from high school or with fewer than 15 semester credits of college coursework. Undergraduate and professional program scholarships are provided, and admission to the professional veterinary medical program is guaranteed upon successful completion of the undergraduate requirements. Mentoring, support services, and summer jobs are also provided.

Eligibility: students who can contribute to the diversity of the program and campus and/or who have a disadvantaged background (economic, cultural, or social). Students must be high-school graduates with fewer than 15 semester credits of college coursework. Selection is competitive. There are 5 positions per year for incoming freshman undergraduate students.

Program dates: begins fall semester; applications available January 1; application deadline March 15.

Contact: College of Veterinary Medicine and Biomedical Sciences, W100 Anatomy, Colorado State University, Fort Collins CO 80523; telephone: (970) 491-7052.

Sponsorship: College of Veterinary Medicine and Biomedical Sciences, Colorado State University, and the U.S. Department of Agriculture.

Cornell University

Program: State University of New York Graduate Underrepresented Minority Fellowships

Description: all matriculating underrepresented minorities are eligible (not restricted by state residency). Minority fellowships include a stipend.

Contact: Director of Financial Aid, College of Veterinary Medicine, S1-006 Schurman Hall, Cornell University, Ithaca NY 14853-6401; telephone (607) 253-3766.

Program: Regents Professional Opportunities Scholarships

Description: a financial assistance program for New York residents who are underrepresented minorities. Must agree to work in New York for a time after graduation.

Contact: Director of Financial Aid, College of Veterinary Medicine, S1-006 Schurman Hall, Cornell University, Ithaca NY 14853-6401; telephone (607) 253-3766.

University of Illinois

Program: Multicultural Fellowhips

Description: to enhance the diversity of the student body and the profession, two $8,000 multicultural fellowships will be available to members of the incoming class. Fellowships are good for four years. Recipients must remain in good academic standing and work with the Office of Academic and Student Affairs with recruiting efforts.

Michigan State University

Program: Vetward Bound Program

Description: Vetward Bound offers 5 levels of programming, each with its own eligibility requirements. Students from high school through prematriculants into the professional program are provided a review of basic science content, research and/or clinical experience, preparation for the GRE and MCAT, veterinary experience, study strategy development, and field experiences. Placement in a specific level is determined by program staff and is based on educational background.

Eligibility: high school through prematriculants into the professional degree program.

Program dates: June through August for 5 to 10 weeks, depending on the specific program content.

Contact: Vetward Bound Coordinator, College of Veterinary Medicine, A-136 East Fee Hall, Michigan State University, East Lansing MI 48824-1316; telephone: (517) 355-6521; e-mail: vetbound@cvm.msu.edu.

Mississippi State University

Program: Board of Trustees of State Institutions of Higher Learning Veterinary Medicine Minority Loan/Scholarship Program

Description: a financial assistance program for Mississippi residents who are underrepresented minorities. Must agree to work in Mississippi for at least 3 years following graduation.

Contact: Director of Student Financial Aid, Mississippi Institutions of Higher Learning, 3825 Ridgewood Road, Jackson MS 39211-6453; telephone: (662) 982-6570.

University of Missouri

Program: Explorations in Veterinary Medicine

Description: a 3-week program to give selected high-school junior or senior students an opportunity to observe and assist in veterinary medical research activities and services offered through the Veterinary Medical Diagnostic Laboratory and the Veterinary Medical Teaching Hospital. A stipend is offered for miscellaneous expenses.

Eligibility: educationally or economically disadvantaged high-school junior or senior students.

Program dates: 3 weeks in July.

Contact: Associate Dean, College of Veterinary Medicine, University of Missouri, Columbia MO 65211.

Program: Gateway and Threshold to Veterinary Medicine

Description: 6-week summer programs to give selected college sophomore, junior, or senior students an opportunity to gain experience with faculty researchers and clinicians in the College of Veterinary Medicine. Travel expenses, room, and board are provided. A stipend is also offered for miscellaneous expenses.

Eligibility: educationally or economically disadvantaged college sophomore, junior, and senior students.

Program dates: mid-June into July.

Contact: Associate Dean, College of Veterinary Medicine, University of Missouri, Columbia MO 65211.

North Carolina State University

Program: Minority Presence Grants

Description: this program provides up to $4,000 annually to African-American North Carolina residents attending the College of Veterinary Medicine.

Frequency: annual program.

Contact: Student Services, College of Veterinary Medicine, (919) 513-6205, www.cvm.ncsu.edu.

Program: Native American Incentive Grant

Description: this program provides up to $4,900 annually to Native American North Carolina residents attending the College of Veterinary Medicine.

Frequency: annual program.

Contact: Student Services, College of Veterinary Medicine, (919) 513-6205, www.cvm.ncsu.edu.

Ohio State University

Program: Young Scholars Program

Description: this summer program is offered to seventh- through eleventh-grade students from Ohio. It provides hands-on science activities.

Eligibility: disadvantaged students from Ohio who have been recommended by their faculty as having academic potential.

Program dates: June to August each summer.

Sponsorship: this program is provided for by funds from the State of Ohio and The Ohio State University.

Program: Medical Science Research Initiative

Description: this program is designed to expose gifted minority high-school students and high-school science teachers to research and animal-related activities through linkage with veterinary college faculty. Though research is the major focus of the program, academic instruction is provided to facilitate scientific knowledge relative to veterinary medicine. A poster presentation of the summer's research project is required at the end of this 8-week program.

Eligibility: eleventh- and twelfth-grade students from Ohio who have demon-strated academic success and have indicated veterinary medicine as a career choice; high-school science teachers who set science education as a high priority.

Program dates: June through August.

Contact: Office of Minority Affairs, The Ohio State University, 1800 Cannon Drive, Columbus OH 43210.

Sponsorship: this program is sponsored by a grant from the U.S. Department of Health and Human Services.

Program: Summer Research Opportunity Program

Description: this program is designed to promote the migration of minority undergraduate students into graduate research educational programs by providing them with summer research experiences. The student is provided with his or her individualized research problem by a faculty mentor and expected to carry that research through to publication.

Eligibility: the student must have completed 2 years of college work and have achieved at least a 2.50 cumulative GPA. The student must be an underrepresented minority or economically disadvantaged.

Contact: Graduate School, The Ohio State University, 230 North Oval Mall, Columbus OH 43210.

Sponsorship: this program is sponsored by the Big Ten Consortium for Institutional Studies.

University of Tennessee

Program: Program for African-American High-School Students

Description: provides African-American high-school students with an opportunity to work with veterinarians in their hometowns for 8 weeks during the summer. During 1 week, students will be guests of the College of Veterinary Medicine on the campus of the University of Tennessee, Knoxville.

Eligibility: African-American juniors or seniors who are residents of Tennessee and enrolled in a Tennessee high school. Applicants must have an interest in veterinary medicine as a potential career. Preference will be given to seniors. Students receive an hourly wage for a 40-hour week.

Contact: Associate Dean, University of Tennessee, College of Veterinary Medicine, P.O. Box 1071, Knoxville TN 37901-1071.

Texas A & M University

Program: Biomedical Science Research Experience

Description: gives freshman college students an opportunity to work in a research laboratory.

Eligibility: graduating high-school seniors.

Program dates: early June through early August.

Contact: Associate Director, Biomedical Science, College of Veterinary Medicine, Texas A & M University, College Station TX 77843-4465; telephone: (409) 845-4941.

Program: Veterinary Enrichment Camp
Description: 3-day program for 40 high-school students.
Eligibility: high-school sophomore, junior, or senior.
Program dates: June.
Contact: Associate Director, Biomedical Science, College of Veterinary Medicine, Texas A & M University, College Station TX 77843-4465; telephone: (409) 845-4941.

Tuskegee University

Program: Health Careers Opportunity Program
Description: this 8-week preadmission activity is designed to facilitate the entry of "at risk" students and provide the skills necessary for successful transition to the professional school.
Eligibility: participation is targeted to minority and disadvantaged students who have completed at least 2 years of college and all preveterinary prerequisites. Participation is restricted to persons who have applied to the College of Veterinary Medicine, Nursing, and Allied Health and who have been selected by the Veterinary Admissions Committee to attend the program.
Program dates: summer before matriculation.
Contact: Assistant Dean, College of Veterinary Medicine, Nursing, and Allied Health, Tuskegee University, Tuskegee AL 36088.
Sponsorship: this program is sponsored by a grant from the U.S. Department of Health and Human Services.

Program: Veterinary Science Training, Education and Preparation Institutes for Minority Students (Vet-Step I and II)
Description: Consists of 2 one-week programs designed to encourage high-achieving minority students to consider veterinary medicine as a career choice. Held in mid-July, the program offers students progressive learning experiences in reading comprehension, note-taking, medical vocabulary, etc. Vet-Step II accepts high-school seniors and those students who have participated in Vet-Step I. The program is sponsored by the U.S. Department of Health and Human Services.
Eligibility: Vet-Step I accepts 25 students from grades 10 and 11; Vet-Step II accepts students from Vet-Step I and from grade 12. Minority high-school honor students interested in the biomedical sciences are eligible to apply.
Contact: Coordinator, Vet-Step Program, College of Veterinary Medicine, Nursing, and Allied Health, Tuskegee University, Tuskegee AL 36088.

Virginia-Maryland Regional College

Program: Minority Summer Research Program — Blacksburg

Description: a 10-week program providing opportunities to conduct scientific research; participate in clinical rotations within the veterinary teaching hospital; improve leadership, public speaking, and self-marketing skills; attend GRE preparatory classes; and learn about admission into graduate/professional school.

Contact: Admissions Office at Blacksburg campus.

Program: Summer Research Apprenticeship Program — College Park

Description: a summer research program providing research experience to veterinary and preveterinary students from diverse backgrounds, including economic hardship and underrepresented racial/ethnic groups. Projects may include assisting in the planning, preparation, and data collection for controlled experiments, clinical trials, or epidemiological investigations; researching disease processes; and performing literature searches.

Contact: Admissions Office at College Park campus.

Scholarship Opportunities: a limited number of scholarships are available to assist minority DVM students.

Washington State University

Program: Short-Term Research Training Program for Veterinary Students

Description: a 3-month summer program designed to promote interest in research by veterinary students. Emphasis is on a hands-on research project supervised by a faculty member with a research program. Stipends are provided.

Eligibility: Washington-Oregon-Idaho program veterinary students or ethnic minority veterinary students from other North American colleges of veterinary medicine.

Program dates: 3 months in the summer dependent upon the summer vacation of the College of Veterinary Medicine in which the veterinary student is enrolled.

Contact: Department of Veterinary Microbiology and Pathology, Washington State University, Pullman WA 99164-7040.

Sponsorship: The National Center for Research Resources.

University of Wisconsin

Program: Pre-College Enrollment Opportunity Program for Learning Excellence (PEOPLE)

Description: this program began in the summer of 1999 as a partnership between the Milwaukee Public Schools and the UW-Madison with a group of students who had just completed the ninth grade. New classes will be added each year, expanding to Madison area schools. The program is designed with a precollege track and a bridge program to undergraduate work and continues through a student's undergraduate career at University of Wisconsin-Madison. The main purposes are to promote academic preparation, increase enrollment in postsecondary institutions, and improve retention and graduation rates of minority students.

Eligibility: students of one or more of the following ethnic heritages: African American, American Indian, Asian American, Hispanic/Latino. Other eligibility factors include economic disadvantage and current enrollment in or commitment to a college preparatory curriculum track.

Program dates: June–July summer residential programs and year-round nonresidential programs.

Contact: Assistant Vice Chancellor, 117 Bascom Hall, University of Wisconsin-Madison, Madison, WI 53706; or Associate Director, University of Wisconsin-Madison Undergraduate Admissions, Armory and Gymnasium, 716 Langdon Street, Madison, WI 53706.

Program: University of Wisconsin-Madison NASA Sharp Plus Program

Description: the NASA Sharp Plus Program is a research-based mentorship program that is jointly sponsored by Quality Education for Minorities (QEM) and the National Aeronautics and Space Administration (NASA). It is an 8-week residential precollege program designed to increase the participation and success rates of students from minority groups that are historically underrepresented in mathematics and sciences. Students are matched with mentors (professors and research scientists) who are currently engaged in scientific research at the university or in an industrial setting.

Eligibility: an applicant must be a U.S. citizen or national, at least 16 years of age, and have completed at least the tenth grade by the start of the program; have completed at least one semester of algebra and geometry and at least one year of biology, chemistry, or physics with a grade of B or better in each of these courses; speak and write English at a level that does not require significant assistance; and be committed to full participation throughout the 8-week program.

Program dates: June–August

Contact: Assistant Vice Chancellor, Room 117 Bascom Hall, University of Wisconsin-Madison, Madison, WI 53706; or Program Coordinator, University of Wisconsin-Madison Medical School, 1140C Medical Science Center, Madison, WI 53706

Scholarships: the School of Veterinary Medicine has a scholarship and other support funding available for preferred students. A portion of those funds come from private donors earmarked specifically for underrepresented groups and individuals who have experienced long-term disadvantages. Please contact the School of Veterinary Medicine if you have questions about these funds.

Financial Aid Information

Financing your veterinary medical education requires careful planning, good money management skills, and a willingness to make short-term sacrifices to achieve long-range goals.

Many of you will apply for and receive some type of financial assistance during your undergraduate education. This will help you become somewhat familiar with the process, and to know that the rules and regulations governing programs can and do change periodically.

As a professional student, you will be entering a partnership with the financial aid office, which will require you to complete the appropriate financial aid forms accurately, meet required deadlines, and submit any additional information that may be requested. In return, the financial aid office will determine your aid eligibility and make awards based on the available programs. Your financial aid eligibility takes into account the cost of your education minus any other available resources. Amounts of assistance and the school policies for awarding assistance vary from one veterinary medical school to another and from year to year.

Any questions or concerns that you may have about this topic need to be directed to each of the appropriate financial aid offices to ensure that you receive accurate information and guidance.

Financing Your Veterinary Medical Education

Your education is one of the biggest investments you will make in your lifetime, and one of your most important goals should be to maximize the return on all of your investments. To reach this goal, you must take an active role in managing your financial resources. You need to understand and implement good financial practices. To get you started, here are some good financial habits you should adopt:

- Do not use credit cards to extend your lifestyle. Deciding not to use credit cards except in emergencies is one of the most important decisions you can make, and one that will reduce your stress while you are pursuing your education.

- Budget your money just as carefully as you budget your time. Contact a financial aid administrator to help you set up a budget that will be easy to follow.

- Distinguish between wants and needs. Before you make any purchase, you should ask yourself, "Do I need this, or do I want it?"

- Be a well-informed borrower. If you have not previously taken an active role in understanding the differences between various student loan programs, now is the time to do it. You need to know these differences in order to avoid high-interest loans and to borrow wisely.

- Borrow the minimum amount necessary in order to maximize the return on your educational investment.

- Be thrifty. Live as cheaply as you can. Remember, you are a student. You'll enjoy a more comfortable lifestyle once you are a DVM.

- Pay any interest that accrues on student loans if you can afford to do so, rather than let the interest accrue and capitalize. Any amount you pay while you're a student will save you money once you enter repayment.

What is the most important piece of advice for making the most of your educational investment? Don't live the lifestyle of a DVM until you have completed your education. Get in the habit of being thrifty. If you live like a DVM while you are in school, you may have to live like a student when you are a DVM.

Federal Loan Programs

	Subsidized Stafford Loan	Unsubsidized Stafford Loan
Lender	Financial or credit institution or eligible school	Financial or credit institution or eligible school
Financial Need	Yes	No
Citizenship Requirement	U.S. Citizen, U.S. National or U.S. Permanent Resident	U.S. Citizen, U.S. National or U.S. Permanent Resident
Borrowing Limits	$8,500/year; $65,500 aggregate undergraduate and graduate	Cost of attendance minus other aid; $189,125 aggregate undergraduate and graduate, less the Subsidized Stafford Loan Total
Interest Rate	Variable; capped at 8.25%	Variable; capped at 8.25%
Interest Accrues School	No	Yes
Deferments	No	Yes
Grace Period	No	Yes

Perkins Loan	Health Professions Student Loan	Loan for Disadvantaged Students
Veterinary Medicine Financial Aid Office	Veterinary Medicine Financial Aid Office	Veterinary Medicine Financial Aid Office
Yes	Yes	Yes
U.S. Citizen, U.S. National or U.S. Permanent Resident	U.S. Citizen, U.S. National or U.S. Permanent Resident	U.S. Citizen, U.S. National or U.S. Permanent Resident
$6,000/year; $40,000 aggregate undergraduate and graduate	Cost of attendance	Cost of attendance
5%	5%	5%
No	No	No
No	No	No
No	No	No

Information about Standardized Tests

Most veterinary medical colleges require one or more standardized tests: the Medical College Admission Test (MCAT), Veterinary College Admission Test (VCAT), or Graduate Record Examination (GRE). For further information regarding test dates and registration procedures, contact the testing agencies listed below:

GRE   Graduate Record Examination
P.O. Box 6000
Princeton NJ 08541-6000
(609) 771-7670 (Princeton, N.J.)
also: (510) 654-1200 (Oakland, Calif.)
Individual School codes: see GRE booklet

MCAT   Medical College Admission Test
MCAT Program Office
P.O. Box 4056
Iowa City IA 52243
(319) 337-1357
VMCAS code 900

VCAT   The Psychological Corporation
Veterinary College Admission Test
555 Academic Court
San Antonio TX 78204
(210) 921-8794
(800) 622-3231
VMCAS code 44

TOEFL   Test of English as a Foreign Language
TOEFL/TSE Services
P.O. Box 6151
Princeton NJ 08541-6151
(609) 771-7100
VMCAS code 4936

Veterinary Medical College Application Service (VMCAS)

The Veterinary Medical College Application Service has been established by the Association of American Veterinary Medical Colleges for applicants wishing to apply to colleges of veterinary medicine in the United States. VMCAS is a centralized application service that provides for the collection, processing, verification, and distribution of applicant data to the participating colleges for their use in the applicant selection process. *This service is a data-processing component of the admissions cycle only; it is in no way a part of the decision-making process, which is the prerogative of the admissions committees at the various colleges of veterinary medicine.*

Application deadlines, prerequisite courses, and other aspects of the selection process differ from college to college. Applicants must pay particular attention to the information and instructions included in the application packet for each of the participating colleges. Questions about the service may be directed to VMCAS, 1101 Vermont Avenue NW, Suite 411, Washington DC 20005-3521. Phone: (202) 682-0750; E-mail: VMCAS@aavmc.org; Web: www.aavmc.org/vmcas. (TTY) (202) 371-0899.

Colleges requiring ALL applicants to submit applications through VMCAS (postmarked by deadline date indicated):

University of California-Davis (Oct 1)
Colorado State University (Oct. 1)
Cornell University (Oct 1)
University of Florida (Oct 1)
University of Georgia (Oct 1)
University of Illinois (Oct 1)
Louisiana State University (Oct 1)
Michigan State University (Oct 1)
University of Minnesota (Oct 1)
North Carolina State University (Oct 1)

Oklahoma State University (Oct 1)
Oregon State University (Nov 1)
University of Pennsylvania (Oct 1)
Purdue University (Oct 1)
University of Tennessee (Nov 1)
Texas A & M University (Oct 1)
Virginia-Maryland Regional College (Oct 1)
Washington State University (Oct 1)
University of Wisconsin (Oct 1)

Colleges requiring only nonresident applicants to submit applications through VMCAS. (Resident applicants are not required to use the service but may do so if applying to multiple VMCAS colleges. Resident applicants applying only to their in-state college should not use this service. Contact your in-state college directly for appropriate application materials.):

Auburn University (Oct 1)   University of Missouri (Oct 1)
Mississippi State University (Oct 1) The Ohio State University (Oct 1)

The service is OPTIONAL for nonresident applicants who wish to apply to the following colleges; however, both nonresident and resident applicants applying to multiple VMCAS colleges may apply through the service. (Resident applicants applying only to their in-state college should not use the service. Contact your in-state college directly for appropriate application materials.)

Iowa State University (Oct 1) Kansas State University (Oct 1)

The service is OPTIONAL for those international (non-Canadian) students who wish to apply to the following colleges. Residents of Canada should not use the service. Contact the college(s) directly for appropriate application materials.

University of Guelph (Dec 1 Canadian; Oct 1 International)
University of Prince Edward Island (Dec 1 Canadian; Oct 1 International)

Colleges requiring students to contact them directly to make application:

UNITED STATES   **CANADA**
Tufts University (Dec 1)   Université de Montréal (Mar 1)
Tuskegee University (Dec 7) University of Saskatchewan (Jan 3)

VETERINARY MEDICAL SCHOOLS IN THE UNITED STATES

Auburn University

Committee on Admissions
College of Veterinary Medicine
217 Goodwin Student Center
Auburn University AL 36849-5536
Telephone: (334) 844-2685
E-mail: admiss@vetmed.auburn.edu
www.vetmed.auburn.edu

The College of Veterinary Medicine at Auburn University is located in south central Alabama on Interstate 85 between Montgomery and Atlanta. The university is known for its friendly small-campus atmosphere despite having more than 21,000 students.

Veterinary medicine began as a department at Auburn in 1892 and became a college in 1907. Today it is situated on 240 acres one mile from the main Auburn campus. In addition, the college has a 700-acre research farm five miles from its campus. The college is fully accredited by the American Veterinary Medical Association.

Application Information

Applications available: June

Application deadline: October 1

Application fee: see VMCAS

Institutional application requirements: $35.00 application fee; applicants who have not previously attended Auburn University are also required to submit a university processing fee of $25.00.

Residency implications: priority is given to Alabama residents. Auburn contracts with Kentucky for 34 positions. Up to 10 nonresident students are accepted.

Veterinary Medical College Application Service (VMCAS): required for all nonresident applicants.

Prerequisites for Admission

Course requirements and semester hours

	Written composition[#]	
*	Literature[#]	6
	Fine Arts[#]	3
	Humanities/fine arts elective[#]	6
*	History[#]	3
	Social/behavioral science electives[#]	9
	Mathematics—precalculus with trigonometry[#]	3
	Principles of biology with lab	3
	Animal biology with lab	3
	Fundamentals of chemistry with lab	8
**	Organic chemistry with lab	6
**	Physics	8
	Biochemistry	3
	Science electives (jr. [300] level or above)	6

* *Students must complete a 6-semester-hour sequence either in literature or in history.*
** *Organic chemistry and physics must have been taken within 6 calendar years.*
# *These requirements will be waived if the student has a bachelor's degree.*

Required undergraduate GPA: a minimum grade point average of at least 2.50 on a 4.00 scale is required, with the minimum acceptable grade for required courses being C-minus. Applicants not classified as Alabama residents or contract students must have a minimum 3.00 GPA on a 4.00 scale. The mean grade point average of the most recent entering class was 3.53.

AP credit policy: must appear on official college transcripts and be equivalent to the appropriate college-level coursework.

Course completion deadline: prerequisite courses must be completed by June 15 prior to matriculation.

Standardized examinations: Graduate Record Examination (GRE), general test, is required. The exam must have been taken within the previous 6 calendar years, and no later than October 1 of the year of application.

Additional requirements and considerations
   Animal/veterinary experience
   Recommendations (3 required)
      Academic advisor or faculty member
      Employer
      Veterinarian
   Extracurricular and community service activities

Employment record

Narrative statement of purpose

Neatness of application

Organic chemistry and physics courses must have been completed within the previous 6 calendar years

Summary of Admission Procedure

Timetable

Application deadline: October 1

Date interviews are held: February–March

Date acceptances mailed: March

School begins: August

Deposit (to hold place in class): none required.

Deferments: not considered.

Evaluation criteria

The 3-part admission procedure includes an objective evaluation of academic credentials, a subjective review of personal credentials, and a personal interview by invitation.

1999–2000 admissions summary

		Number of Applicants	Number of New Entrants
Resident		123	46
Contract*		93	34
Nonresident		589	10
	Total:	805	90

Expenses for the 1999–2000 Academic Year

Tuition and fees

Resident	$6,000.00
Nonresident	
Contract*	$6,000.00
Other nonresident	$18,000.00

* For further information, see the listing of contracting states and provinces.

University of California

Office of the Dean — Student Programs
School of Veterinary Medicine
University of California
One Shields Avenue
Davis CA 95616
Telephone: (530) 752-1383
www.ucdavis.edu

The University of California, Davis (UCD) campus is adjacent to the city of Davis, which is 14 miles west of Sacramento, the state capital, and 72 miles northeast of San Francisco. Davis is known as the "city of bicycles." The community is closely tied to the university yet has developed its own recreational, cultural, and community outlets. Winter temperatures are generally mild and rarely fall below freezing. Summers are sunny, hot, and dry. Weather in the spring and fall is the most pleasant in the state. UCD is an outstanding research and training institution with approximately 24,500 undergraduate, graduate, and professional students enrolled in 4 colleges and professional schools (Veterinary Medicine, Medicine, Law, and Management). The educational buildings and research facilities are situated on over 5,200 acres at Davis and 10 off-campus field stations. UCD is the home of the Veterinary Medical Teaching Hospital, the California Regional Primate Research Center, the California Animal Health and Food Safety Laboratory System, the Veterinary Medical Teaching and Research Center, and the Center for Comparative Medicine. There are many innovative programs at UCD with many international students. The school is fully committed to recruiting students with diverse backgrounds.

Application Information

Applications available: May

Application deadline: October 1

Application fee: see VMCAS

Residency implications: priority is given to California residents. California accepts no more than a total of 2 applicants from WICHE states (Alaska, Arizona, Hawaii, Montana, Nevada, New Mexico, North Dakota, Utah, and Wyoming), and California may accept a small number of uniquely qualified nonresident applicants.

34

Veterinary Medical College Application Service (VMCAS): required for all applicants.

Prerequisites for Admission

Course requirements and quarter hours

General chemistry (with laboratory)	15
Organic chemistry (with laboratory)	6
Biochemistry* (bioenergetics and metabolism)	4
Physics	6
Biology and zoology (1 laboratory requirement)	10
Systemic physiology*	5
Vertebrate embryology*	4
Genetics*	4
English composition and additional English	12
Humanities and social sciences	12
Statistics	4

* Upper-division courses equivalent to one semester or one quarter

Note: equivalent courses may vary in units and may also require other prerequisites.

Required undergraduate GPA: a minimum grade point average of 2.50 on a 4.00 scale is required for *both* the required sciences and cumulative college coursework. Applicants admitted in fall 1999 had a mean cumulative GPA of 3.45.

AP credit policy: not available.

Course completion deadline: all prerequisite courses must be completed by the time a student plans to enroll.

Standardized examinations: Graduate Record Examination (GRE), general test, is required. The most recent acceptable GRE test date for applicants entering fall 2001 is September 30, 2000. Date of oldest acceptable scores is October 1995. Average GRE scores for the class admitted in 1999 are verbal 600, quantitative 701, and analytical 724.

Additional requirements and considerations

Veterinary/animal experience
Letters of evaluation (3)
Personal statement of motivation/career goals
Accuracy and neatness of application
Interview/essay

Summary of Admission Procedure

Timetable
   Application deadline: October 1
   Date interviews are held: February to mid-March
   Date acceptances mailed: by April 1
   School begins: early September

Deposit (to hold place in class): none required.

Deferments: not considered.

Evaluation criteria	% weight
Grades	30
Test scores	30
Personal Statement/Essay/Animal and Veterinary Experience/References	20
Interview	20

1999–2000 admissions summary

	Number of Applicants	Number of New Entrants
Resident	526	117
Contract*	85	1
Nonresident	455	4
Total:	1,066	122

Expenses for the 1999–2000 Academic Year

Tuition and fees
Resident	$10,500.00
Nonresident	$20,300.00
Contract student*	$20,300.00

* For further information, see the listing of contracting states and provinces.

Dual-Degree Programs
Combined DVM-graduate degree programs are available.

Colorado State University

Office of the Dean
College of Veterinary Medicine and Biomedical Sciences
Colorado State University
Fort Collins CO 80523-1601
Telephone: (970) 491-7052
E-mail: mstokes@cvmbs.colostate.edu
www.cvmbs.colostate.edu

Colorado State University is located in Fort Collins, a city of about 100,000 in the eastern foothills of the Rocky Mountains about 60 miles north of Denver. Fort Collins has a pleasant climate and offers many cultural and recreational activities. Many of the state's ski areas lie within a short driving distance, making some of the best skiing in the world accessible. The nearby river canyons and mountain parks are beautiful scenic attractions and provide opportunities for hiking, fishing, photography, camping, and biking.

The College of Veterinary Medicine and Biomedical Sciences is composed of 5 major buildings, which house the departments of anatomy and neurobiology, microbiology, environmental health, pathology, physiology, and radiological health sciences. The Veterinary Teaching Hospital, one of the world's largest and best-equipped, houses the clinical sciences department. The hospital attracts a large caseload and offers students a wide variety of clinical experiences.

Application Information

Applications available: May

Application deadline: October 1

Application fee: see VMCAS

Institutional application requirements: $40.00 application fee

Residency implications: positions are allocated as follows: Colorado 75, WICHE contracts (Arizona 17, Hawaii 5, Montana 7, Nevada 4, New Mexico 10, North Dakota 1, Utah 6, Wyoming 4), and nonsponsored 10-20. WICHE students must be certified by their states. Nonsponsored students can be from any state or country.

Veterinary Medical College Application Service (VMCAS): required for all applicants.

Prerequisites for Admission

Course requirements and semester hours

Laboratory associated with a biology course	1
Genetics	3
Laboratory associated with a chemistry course	1
Biochemistry	3
Physics (with laboratory)	4
Statistics/biostatistics	3
English composition	3
Social sciences and humanities	12
Electives	38

Required undergraduate GPA: the mean GPA for the 1999 matriculated class was 3.68 on a 4.00 scale.

AP credit policy: must appear on official college transcripts.

Course completion deadline: transcripts with final grades, including all required courses, must be received by July 15 prior to matriculation.

Standardized examinations: Graduate Record Examination (GRE), general test, is required and must be taken within the last five years prior to application. Scores must be received by October 1, 2000. Mean GRE scores for the 1999 matriculated class were verbal 521, quantitative 609, analytical 627.

Additional requirements and considerations
Animal/veterinary/unique work experience
Recommendations (3 preferred)
    Academic (academic advisor or college professor)
    Employer
    Veterinarian
Essay
Extracurricular and community service activities, leadership
Quality of academic program (course load, challenging curriculum, honors)
Contributions to diversity, extenuating circumstances

Summary of Admission Procedure

Timetable
Application deadline: October 1
Date interviews are held: early February
School begins: late August

Deposit (to hold place in class): none required.

Deferments: not considered.

Evaluation criteria
Grades, quality of academic program
GRE scores
Animal/veterinary/other work experience
Activities & achievements, community service
Essay
Letters of recommendation
Interview (Colorado only)

1999–2000 admissions summary

	Number of Applicants	*Number of New Entrants*
Sponsored	346	75
Sponsored (WICHE)*	200	41
Nonsponsored	299	17
Total:	845	133

Expenses for the 1999–2000 Academic Year

Tuition and fees (first-year students only)
Sponsored $8,640.00
Nonsponsored $29,242.00

* For further information, see the listing of contracting states and provinces.

Dual-Degree Programs

Combined DVM–graduate degree programs are available.

Cornell University

Office of DVM Admissions
College of Veterinary Medicine
S1-006 Schurman Hall
Cornell University
Ithaca, NY 14853-6401
Telephone: (607) 253-3700
E-mail: vet_admissions@cornell.edu
www.vet.cornell.edu

Cornell is located in Ithaca, a city of about 30,000 in the Finger Lakes region of upstate New York, a beautiful area of rolling hills, deep valleys, scenic gorges, and clear lakes. The university's 740-acre campus is bounded on two sides by gorges and waterfalls. Open countryside, state parks, and year-round opportunities for outdoor recreation, including excellent sailing, swimming, skiing, hiking, and other activities, are only minutes away.

Ithaca is one hour by air and a four-hour drive from New York City, and other major metropolitan areas are easily accessible. Direct commercial flights connect Ithaca with New York, Boston, Chicago, Pittsburgh, Washington, and other cities.

The tradition of academic excellence, the cultural vigor of a distinguished university, and the magnificent setting create a stimulating environment for graduate study. The college opened a new Veterinary Education Center in 1993 and extensive new clinical and research facilities in 1995.

Application Information

Applications available: May

Application deadline: October 1

Application fee: see VMCAS

Institutional application requirements: $40-65 application fee.

Residency implications: approximately 60 places reserved for New York State residents. The College of Veterinary Medicine at Cornell currently has contracts with New Hampshire, New Jersey, and Puerto Rico. There are a variable number of places available for nonresidents.

Veterinary Medical College Application Service (VMCAS): required for all applicants.

Prerequisites for Admission

Course requirements and semester hours

English composition*	6
Biology or zoology, full year with laboratory	6
Physics, full year with laboratory	6
Inorganic (general) chemistry, full year with laboratory	6
Organic chemistry, full year with laboratory	6
Biochemistry	4
General microbiology, with laboratory	3
Electives	53

* Three credits may be satisfied by a course in public speaking.

All prerequisites must have a letter grade of "C-" or better. Advanced placement credits will not be accepted for courses other than physics and inorganic chemistry.

Required undergraduate GPA: Cornell does not have a GPA requirement, but the grade range of those admitted tends to be 3.00–4.00. The median GPA for the class of 2003 was 3.60.

AP credit policy: not available.

Course completion deadline: all but 12 credits of the prerequisite coursework should be completed at the time of application, with at least one semester of any two-semester series completed. Any outstanding prerequisites must be completed by the end of the spring term prior to matriculation.

Standardized examinations: Graduate Record Examination (GRE), general test, is required. The most recent acceptable test date for applicants to the class of 2004 is the September 30, 2000 exam. The class of 2003 had a median score of 1340 (verbal 630 and quantitative 710). Test scores older than 5 years will not be accepted.

Additional requirements and considerations

    Animal/veterinary experience, knowledge, and motivation
    Recommendations/evaluations (3 required)
        Academic advisor
        Animal-experience employers
        Nonveterinary work-related experiences
    Essay
    Extracurricular and/or community service activities
    Demonstrated leadership skills
    Quality of academic program

Summary of Admission Procedure

Timetable
Application deadline: October 1
Information sessions at the college: February–March
Date acceptance mailed: February
School begins: late August

Deposit (to hold place in class): $500.00.

Deferments: considered on an individual basis, but ordinarily granted only for illness or other problem beyond the voluntary control of the applicant.

Evaluation criteria
The admission procedure consists of 2 phases: an objective evaluation of academic credentials and a subjective review of the overall application.

	% weight
Grades	30
Test scores	30
Animal/veterinary experience	20
References, essay, quality of academic program, and nonacademic activities	20

1999–2000 admissions summary

	Number of Applicants	*Number of New Entrants*
Resident	274	50
Contract*	80	4
Nonresident	898	26
Total:	1,252	80

Expenses for the 1999–2000 Academic Year

Tuition and fees

Resident	$14,900.00
Nonresident	
Contract student*	$14,900.00
Other nonresident	$20,100.00

* For further information, see the listing of contracting states and provinces.

Dual-Degree Programs

Combined DVM-graduate degree programs are available.

Early Admission Program

The Leadership Training Program targets gifted first-year veterinary medical students who are potential leaders in the profession. The major objective of the program is to acquaint students with veterinary medical career opportunities in academic institutions, government, and industry. The program also encourages networking among the participants. Fellowships are available. For further information, contact: Graduate Education Coordinator, Schurman Hall, Cornell University, Ithaca, NY 14853; telephone (607) 253-3720.

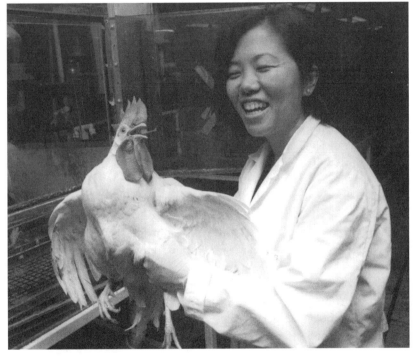

A student specializing in avian medicine examines a chicken as part of her study. Photo by Joey Rodgers, courtesy University of Georgia College of Veterinary Medicine.

University of Florida

College of Veterinary Medicine
Admissions Office
P.O. Box 100125
University of Florida
Gainesville FL 32610-0125
Telephone: (352) 392-4700, ext. 5300
E-mail: henryt@mail.vetmed.ufl.edu
www.vetmed.ufl.edu

The University of Florida is located in Gainesville, a college town of approximately 100,000 in north central Florida, midway between the Gulf of Mexico and the Atlantic Ocean. Changes in season are marked, but winters are mild and permit year-round participation in outdoor activities.

The university accommodates about 40,000+ students with programs in almost all disciplines. The College of Veterinary Medicine is a component of the Institute of Food and Agriculture Sciences (which also includes Agriculture and Forest Resources and Conservation). It is also one of 6 colleges affiliated with the Health Science Center (the other 5 are Dentistry, Health-related Professions, Medicine, Nursing, and Pharmacy).

The veterinary curriculum is a 9-semester program consisting of core curriculum and elective experiences. The core provides the body of knowledge and skills common to all veterinarians. The first 4 semesters concentrate primarily on basic medical sciences. Students are additionally introduced to physical diagnosis, radiology, and clinical problems during these years. The core also includes experience in each of the clinical areas. Elective areas of concentration permit students to investigate further the aspects of both basic and clinical sciences most relevant to their interests.

Application Information

Applications available: May

Application deadline: October 1

Application fee: see VMCAS

Residency implications: priority is given to Florida residents, and Florida has no contractual agreements. Nonresidents are considered in very limited numbers (not more than 15% of any entering class).

Veterinary Medical College Application Service (VMCAS): required for all applicants.

Prerequisites for Admission

Course requirements and semester hours

Biology (general, genetics, microbiology)	15
Chemistry (inorganic, organic, biochemistry)	19
Physics	8
Mathematics (calculus, statistics)	6
Animal Science (introduction to animal science, animal nutrition)	6
Humanities	9
Social sciences	6
English (2 courses in English composition)	6
Electives	at least 5

Required undergraduate GPA: a minimum GPA of 2.75 on a 4.00 scale. The class of 2003 had an overall mean science prerequisite GPA of 3.41.

AP credit policy: must appear on official college transcripts and be equivalent to the appropriate college-level coursework.

Course completion deadline: prerequisite courses must be completed by the end of the spring term prior to admission.

Standardized examinations: Graduate Record Examination (GRE) is required. October 2000 is the most recent acceptable test date for applicants to the class of 2004. Mean score for the class of 2003 was 1187.

Additional requirements and considerations

Animal/veterinary experience
Recommendations/evaluations (3 required)
    Personal
    Veterinarian
    Academic advisor
Honors and awards received
Extracurricular activities
Essay

Summary of Admission Procedure

Timetable
    Application deadline: October 1
    Date interviews are held: March
    Date acceptances mailed: April 1
    School begins: mid-August

Deposit (to hold place in class): none required.

Deferments: considered on an individual basis.

Evaluation criteria
The admission procedure consists of 3 parts: each applicant's file is reviewed; selected applicants are each interviewed for about 20 minutes by 3 faculty members; final selection of new class takes place.

1999–2000 admissions summary

		Number of Applicants	Number of New Entrants
Resident		245	73
Contract		N/A	N/A
Nonresident		566	7
	Total:	811	80

Expenses for the 1999–2000 Academic Year

Tuition and fees
    Resident $8,211.00
    Nonresident $21,748.00

University of Georgia

Office for Academic Affairs
College of Veterinary Medicine
University of Georgia
Athens GA 30602-7372
Telephone: (706) 542-5728
E-mail: ywilson@calc.vet.uga.edu
www.vet.uga.edu

The University of Georgia is located in Athens-Clarke County, with a population of 86,000. Georgia's "Classic City" is a prospering community that reflects the charm of the Old South while growing in culture and industry. Athens is just over an hour away from the north Georgia mountains and the metropolitan area of Atlanta, and just over 5 hours away from the Atlantic coast.

In 1785, Georgia became the first state to grant a charter for a state-supported university. In 1801 the first students came to the newly formed frontier town of Athens. The University of Georgia has grown into an institution with 13 schools and colleges and more than 2,700 faculty members and 30,000 students.

Application Information

Applications available: May

Application deadline: October 1

Application fee: see VMCAS

Institutional application requirements: $30.00 application fee

Residency implications: Georgia retains up to 23 positions for contract students. Contracts are with South Carolina (maximum 17) and West Virginia (maximum 6). The balance of those admitted are residents of Georgia or nonresident, noncontract applicants.

Veterinary Medical College Application Service (VMCAS): required for all applicants.

47

Prerequisites for Admission

Course requirements and semester hours

English	6
Humanities and social studies	14
General biology	8
Advanced biological science	8
Chemistry	
Inorganic	8
Organic	8
Physics	8
Biochemistry	3

Required undergraduate GPA: cumulative GPA of 3.00 or greater on a 4.00 scale *or* a combined score on the GRE verbal and quantitative sections of 1200 or greater.

AP credit policy: must appear on official college transcripts and be equivalent to the appropriate college-level coursework.

Course completion deadline: prerequisite courses must be completed by the end of the spring term preceding entry.

Standardized examinations: Graduate Record Examination (GRE), general test, and the biology subject test must be completed within the 3 years immediately preceding the deadline for receipt of applications (October 1). Test scores must be received by February 1 after the October 1 application deadline.

Additional requirements and considerations
>   Animal experience
>   Background for veterinary medicine
>   Recommendations/evaluations (3 required)
>   Academic advisor/faculty member (required for graduate students)
>   Employer
>   Veterinarian
>   Essay

Summary of Admission Procedure

Timetable
>   Application deadline: October 1
>   Date acceptances mailed: late March
>   School begins: late August

Deposit (to hold place in class): $100.00; $500.00 for nonresident, noncontract students.

Deferments: one-year deferments considered for reasons such as completing a degree or for health problems.

Evaluation criteria
The admissions procedure includes a file evaluation. There are no interviews, but applicants are invited to a college orientation.

Academic performance
Standardized test scores
Animal/veterinary experience
References
Employment history
Narrative statement
Extracurricular activities

1999-2000 admissions summary

		Number of Applicants	Number Accepted
Resident		233	58
Contract*		87	23
Nonresident		500	5
	Total:	820	86

Expenses for the 1999-2000 Academic Year

Tuition and fees (approximate)
Resident	$6,462.00
Nonresident	
Contract*	$6,462.00
Nonresident	$18,262.00

* For further information, see the listing of contracting states and provinces.

University of Illinois

Office of Academic and Student Affairs
College of Veterinary Medicine
University of Illinois at Urbana-Champaign
2271G Veterinary Medicine Basic Sciences Bldg.
2001 South Lincoln Avenue
Urbana IL 61802
Telephone: (217) 333-1192
E-mail: admissions@cvm.uiuc.edu
www.cvm.uiuc.edu

The University of Illinois is in Urbana-Champaign, a community of about 100,000 people located 140 miles south of Chicago. It is served by 4 airlines, 3 interstate highways, bus, and rail. The twin cities and university make a pleasant community with easy access to all areas and facilities. The university has about 35,000 students and more than 11,000 faculty and staff members. It is known for its high-quality academic programs and its exceptional resources and facilities. The university library has the largest collection of any public university and ranks third among all U.S. academic libraries. The university also has outstanding cultural and sports facilities and activities.

The College of Veterinary Medicine is located at the south edge of the campus in a large physical plant built in phases since 1971. In addition to approximately 380 students, the college has about 100 graduate students plus a full complement of residents and interns. There are more than 100 full-time faculty with research interests in a variety of biomedical sciences and clinical areas. This research activity allows a variety of interactions and employment for students. The college also offers students a stimulating core-elective curriculum to prepare for a career in almost any area of the profession.

Application Information

Applications available: May

Application deadline: October 1

Application fee: see VMCAS

Institutional application requirements: $40.00 (U.S. citizens) and $50.00 (international students) application fee

Residency implications: priority is given to approximately 80 Illinois residents; approximately 20 nonresident positions.

50

Veterinary Medical College Application Service (VMCAS): required for all applicants.

Prerequisites for Admission

The academic requirements for application to the College of Veterinary Medicine can be met through one of two pathways: Plan A or Plan B. Those considering a career in veterinary medicine should have a good foundation in biological sciences and chemistry, including *biochemistry*, and should consider the specific courses listed in Plan A as a minimum knowledge base for success in the curriculum. In addition, a course or courses concerning livestock production and animal ethology are highly desirable for all students. Those seeking a career in veterinary medicine related to agriculture should consider additional background in nutrition, livestock management, and the economics of production by working toward a degree in animal science prior to admission to veterinary school.

Plan A

BS or BA degree in any major field of study from an accredited college or university including the following courses (equivalent in content to those required for students majoring in biological sciences):

a. 8 semester hours of biological sciences with laboratories
b. 16 semester hours of chemical sciences, including organic and biochemistry, with laboratories in inorganic and organic chemistry
c. 8 semester hours of physics with laboratories

Plan B

Those applying without a bachelor's degree are required to present at least 60 semester hours from an accredited college or university, including 40 hours of science courses. The minimum course requirements under Plan B are:

a. 8 semester hours of biological sciences with laboratories
b. 16 semester hours of chemical sciences, including organic and biochemistry, with laboratories in inorganic and organic chemistry
c. 8 semester hours of physics with laboratories
d. 3 semester hours of English composition and an additional 3 hours of English composition and/or speech
e. 12 semester hours of humanities and social sciences
f. 10 semester hours of junior/senior-level courses in addition to the requirements listed above

Required undergraduate GPA: a minimum cumulative GPA of 2.75 and a minimum science GPA of 2.75 on a 4.00 scale are required. The mean cumulative GPA for students invited to interview in 1999 was 3.67, mean science GPA was 3.63, and mean GRE score was 72 (percentile).

AP credit policy: not available.

Standardized examinations: Graduate Record Examination (GRE), general test, is required. Test must be taken by October 1 of the year of application, and scores may be no older than two years.

Additional requirements and considerations
    Animal veterinary knowledge, motivation, and experience
    Recommendations/evaluations
        Animal- and veterinary-experience employer
        Academic advisor
    Evidence of leadership, initiative, and responsibility
    Rigor of academic preparation

Summary of Admission Procedure

Timetable
    Application deadline: October 1
    Informational program and required interviews: early March
    Date acceptances mailed: mid-March
    School begins: late August

Deposit (to hold place in class): none required.

Deferments: not considered.

Evaluation criteria
A 2-part admission procedure is used. A file evaluation, stressing academic achievement and personal qualities, is followed by a personal interview.

	% weight
Test scores	20
Science GPA	25
Cumulative GPA	15
Subjective points:	30
academic rigor, veterinary experience, animal experience, evidence of leadership ability, and letters of evaluation.	
Interview	10

1999–2000 admissions summary

	Number of Applicants	*Number of New Entrants*
Resident	248	83
Nonresident	822	21
Total:	1,070	104

Expenses for the 2000-2001 Academic Year

Tuition and fees
Resident	$10,090.00
Nonresident	$24,872.00

Dual-Degree Programs

Combined DVM-graduate degree programs are available.

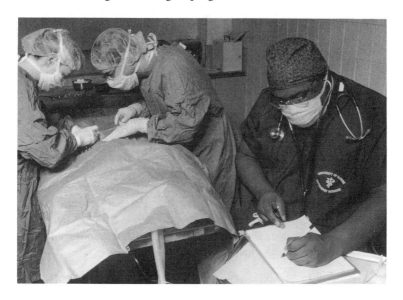

Students in the junior surgery program at the University of Illinois College of Veterinary Medicine spay and neuter animals for local humane societies. Photo by Lil Morales, courtesy University of Illinois College of Veterinary Medicine.

Iowa State University

Office of Admissions
Room 100 Alumni Hall
Iowa State University
Ames IA 50011
Telephone: (515) 294-5836
Toll free outside Iowa: (800) 262-3810
www.vetmed.iastate.edu

The Iowa State University College of Veterinary Medicine is located in the heart of one of the world's most intensive livestock-producing areas, which provides diverse food-animal clinical and diagnostic cases. A nearby metropolitan area and a regionally recognized referral veterinary hospital provide experience in companion-animal medicine and surgery. A racetrack is located near the college and provides an increasing number of challenging equine patients.

A strong basic science education during the first 2 years prepares veterinary students for a wide range of clinical experiences during the last 2 years. The College of Veterinary Medicine provides education in a wide variety of animal species and disciplines and allows fourth-year students to spend time with private practitioners, other colleges, research facilities, and in other educational experiences. Opportunities for research exist in the outstanding research programs in neurobiology, immunobiology, infectious diseases, and numerous other areas, and the nearby National Animal Disease Center and the National Veterinary Services Laboratories provide additional opportunities. The world's premier State Diagnostic Laboratory is part of the college and provides students with experience that is unmatched by any other veterinary college in the world. Graduates are highly sought after and can typically choose among 5 or 6 job offers. A career development and placement service is also provided.

Application Information

Applications available: July

Application deadline: October 1

Application fee: $20.00

Institutional application requirements: request application packet from Iowa State University Office of Admissions, and submit required information no later than stated deadlines.

Residency implications: priority is given to Iowa residents for approximately 60 positions. Iowa contracts on a year-to-year basis with New Jersey, North Dakota, and South Dakota. Remaining positions are available for residents of noncontract states or international students.

Veterinary Medical College Application Service (VMCAS): optional for all applicants.

Prerequisites for Admission

Course requirements and semester hours

English composition	6
General chemistry (with laboratory)	8
Organic chemistry (with laboratory)	7
Biochemistry	3
Physics	8
Biology	8
Genetics	3
Mammalian anatomy and/or physiology	3
Speech	3
Arts, humanities, or social sciences	9
Electives	8

Required undergraduate GPA: the minimum GPA required by Iowa State University is 2.50 on a 4.00 scale. The most recent entering class had a mean GPA of 3.57 with a range of 3.04 to 4.00.

AP credit policy: must be documented by original scores submitted to the university, and must meet the university's minimum requirement in the appropriate subject area.

Course completion deadline: prerequisite courses must be completed by June 15 prior to matriculation.

Standardized examinations: Graduate Record Examination (GRE), general test, is required.

Additional requirements and considerations
Recommendations (3 required). Academic advisors, veterinarians, and employers are suggested.

Summary of Admission Procedure

Timetable
  Application deadline: October 1
  Date acceptances mailed: March 15
  School begins: late August

Deposit (to hold place in class): $250.00

Deferments: not considered.

Evaluation criteria
Personal interviews are not conducted. The admission procedure consists of a review of each candidate's application and qualifications:

1. Academic factors include grades, test scores, and degrees earned.
2. Nonacademic factors include personal statement, experience, recommendations, and personal development activities.

1999–2000 admissions summary

		Number of Applicants	Number of New Entrants
Resident		128	62
Contract*		93	24
Nonresident		866	14
	Total:	1,087	100

Expenses for the 1999–2000 Academic Year

Tuition and fees
  Resident $6,082.00
  Nonresident
    Contract*   varies by contract
    Other nonresident $17,328.00

* For further information, see the listing of contracting states and provinces.

Dual-Degree Programs

Combined DVM-graduate degree programs are available.

Kansas State University

Office of Admissions
College of Veterinary Medicine
101 Trotter Hall
1700 Denison Avenue
Kansas State University
Manhattan KS 66506-5601
Telephone: (785) 532-4335
Fax: (785) 532-4850
E-mail: admit@vet.ksu.edu
www.vet.ksu.edu

Kansas State University in Manhattan, Kansas, is located 125 miles west of Kansas City near Interstate 70. With a population of about 60,000 including KSU, Manhattan is in an area surrounded by many historical points of interest in a rich agricultural area of north central Kansas. Recreational activities abound in Manhattan and the surrounding area with fishing, boating, camping, and hunting among the favorites. Sporting events, theater, concerts, and excellent parks contribute to the many activities available. Kansans enjoy the 4 seasons, each of which brings its own special activities and events.

Kansas State University is on a beautiful 664-acre campus. The College of Veterinary Medicine opened in 1905. It is located on 80 acres just north of the main campus in 3 interconnected buildings.

Application Information

Applications available: July

Application deadline: October 1

Application fee: $50.00

Institutional application requirements: request supplemented application packet from the Office of Admissions prior to September 15.

Residency implications: priority is given to Kansas residents; to be eligible to be in the Kansas pool of applicants, the applicant must be a Kansas resident for tuition purposes at the time of application. Kansas contracts with Nebraska. Kansas accepts about 25 nonresident, noncontract students per year.

Veterinary Medical College Application Service (VMCAS): optional for all applicants.

Prerequisites for Admission

Course Requirements and Semester Hours

Expository writing I and II	6
Public speaking	2
Chemistry I and II	8
General organic chemistry, with laboratory	5
General biochemistry, with laboratory	5
Physics I and II	8
Principles of biology or general zoology	4
Mammalian embryology, with laboratory, or developmental biology *	4
Microbiology, with laboratory	4
Animal genetics or general genetics	3
Social sciences and /or humanities	12
Electives	9

* If a course in embryology or developmental biology is not offered at the school you are attending, please contact the office of the Assistant Dean. Comparative anatomy, reproductive physiology, or an advanced animal biology course may be approved for substitution.

All science courses must have been taken within six years of the date of enrollment in the professional program.

Required undergraduate GPA: the required GPA is a 2.80 on a 4.00 scale in both the prerequisite courses and the last 45 semester hours of undergraduate work. The most recent entering class had a mean prerequisite science GPA of 3.43.

AP credit policy: must appear on official college transcripts and be equivalent to the appropriate college-level coursework.

Course completion deadline: prerequisite courses must be completed by the end of the spring term of the year in which admission is sought.

Standardized examinations: Graduate Record Examination (GRE), general test, is required by October 1. Nonresident, noncontract applicants having combined scores of less than 1800 are not likely to be interviewed.

Additional requirements and considerations

Animal/veterinary work experience and knowledge

Employment record

3 evaluations required by nonfamily members, one a veterinarian. Other suggested references include academic or preprofessional advisor, professor, or other professional.

Summary of Admission Procedure

Timetable
Application deadline: October 1
Date interviews are held:
    Kansas residents: late December
    Nebraska residents: early February
    Nonresident: early January
Date acceptances mailed: within one month after interview
School begins: mid-August

Deposit (to hold place in class): $100.00 for Kansas and contract state residents, $250.00 for nonresident students.

Deferments: may be granted by Admissions Committee for extraordinary circumstances.

Evaluation criteria
A 4-part admission procedure is used, including evaluation of science grades, evaluation of all 3 GRE scores, assessment of the application and narrative, and a personal interview.

Prerequisite science GPA	30%
Test scores	40%
Interview score including:	30%
References	
Animal/veterinary experience	
Leadership in college and community	
Autobiographical essay	

1999–2000 admissions summary

	Number of Applicants	Number of New Entrants
Resident	120	51
Contract*	79	27
Nonresident	539	22
Total:	738	100

*   For further information, see the listing of contracting states and provinces.

Expenses for the 1999–2000 Academic Year

Tuition and fees (subject to change)

Resident	$5,500.00
Nonresident	
Contract*	$5,500.00
Other nonresident	$17,800.00

* For further information, see the listing of contracting states and provinces.

Dual-Degree Programs

Combined DVM-graduate degree programs are available.

Early Admission Program

The Veterinary Scholars Early Admission Program is designed for those students having a genuine desire to enter the veterinary profession who attend Kansas State University with an ACT score of 29 or greater or a comparable composite SAT score and who complete a successful interview during the fall semester of their freshman year.

Louisiana State University

Office of Veterinary Student Affairs
School of Veterinary Medicine
Louisiana State University
Baton Rouge LA 70803
Telephone: (225) 346-3155
Fax: (225) 346-5706
E-mail: cmiceli@mail.vetmed.lsu.edu
www.vetmed.lsu.edu

The Louisiana State University campus is located in Baton Rouge, which has a population of more than 500,000 and is a major industrial city, a thriving port, and the state's capital. Since it is located on the Mississippi River, Baton Rouge was a target for domination by Spanish, French, and English settlers. The city bears the influence of all 3 cultures and offers a range of choices in everything from food to architectural design. Geographically, Baton Rouge is the center of south Louisiana's main cultural and recreational attractions. Equally distant from New Orleans and the fabled Cajun bayou country, there is an abundance of cultural and outdoor recreational activities. South Louisiana has a balmy climate that encourages lush vegetation and comfortable temperatures year round.

The campus encompasses more than 2,000 acres in the southern part of Baton Rouge and is bordered on the west by the Mississippi River. The Veterinary Medicine Building, occupied in 1978, houses the academic departments, the veterinary library, and the Veterinary Teaching Hospital and clinics. The school is fully accredited by the American Veterinary Medical Association.

Application Information

Applications available: May

Application deadline: October 1

Application fee: see VMCAS

Residency implications: Louisiana contracts with Arkansas (9). Louisiana accepts a limited number of highly qualified nonresident applicants.

Veterinary Medical College Application Service (VMCAS): required for all applicants.

Prerequisites for Admission

Course requirements and semester hours

Biology	8
Microbiology	4
Physics	6
General chemistry	8
Organic chemistry	3
Biochemistry	3
English composition	6
Speech communication	3
Mathematics	5
Electives	20

Required undergraduate GPA: the minimum acceptable GPA for required coursework is 2.50 on a 4.00 scale. The mean GPA of the most recent entering class at the time of acceptance was 3.61.

AP credit policy: must appear on official college transcripts and be equivalent to the appropriate college-level coursework.

Course completion deadline: prerequisite courses must be completed by the end of the spring term preceding matriculation.

Standardized examinations: Medical College Admission Test or Graduate Record Examination, general test, is required. The most recent acceptable test date is early fall of the year of application. The average GRE combined verbal and quantitative score was 1107 for the class of 2003.

Additional requirements and considerations
Animal/veterinary work experience
Motivation, maturity
Demonstrated communication skills
Breadth of interests

Summary of Admission Procedure

Timetable
Application deadline: October 1
Date interviews are held: early March
Date acceptances mailed: late March
School begins: late August

Deposit (to hold place in class): $500.00 for nonresidents.

Deferments: considered.

Evaluation criteria

The approximate components of the evaluation scoring are:

Objective evaluation:

GPA required courses	32%
GPA last 45 hours	20%
Test scores	18%

Subjective evaluation:

Animal/veterinary experience, references (3 required, one by a veterinarian), essay	16%
Personal interview	10%
Committee evaluation	4%

1999–2000 admissions summary

		Number of Applicants	*Number of New Entrants*
Resident		209	66
Contract*		67	10
Nonresident		868	4
	Total:	1,144	80

Expenses for the 2000-2001 Academic Year

Tuition and fees (estimated)

Resident	$6,060.00
Nonresident	
Contract*	$6,060.00
Other nonresident	$18,250.00

* Further information, see the listing of contracting states and provinces.

Michigan State University

Office of Admissions
College of Veterinary Medicine
A-126 East Fee Hall
Michigan State University
East Lansing MI 48824-1316
Telephone: (517) 353-9793; fax: (517) 432-2391; helpline: (800) 496-4678
E-mail: admiss@cvm.msu.edu
www.cvm.msu.edu

Michigan State University's campus is bordered by the city of East Lansing, which offers sidewalk cafes, restaurants, shops, and convenient mass transit. The campus is traversed by the Red Cedar River and has many miles of bike paths and walkways. This park-like setting provides an ideal venue in which MSU's 41,000 students may enjoy outdoor concerts and plays, canoeing, and cross-country skiing. North of the river is the older part of campus. The ivy-covered buildings, some built before the Civil War and listed on the National Register of Historic Places, house 5 colleges, the student union, and 10 residence halls. South of the river are more recent additions to the campus, such as the Wharton Center for Performing Arts, the Jack Breslin Student Events Center, and several intramural sports facilities.

The college is a national leader in state-of-the-art technology and facilities. A lecture hall is equipped with a computer at each of the 116 work stations. These computers are part of a network that links all parts of the Veterinary Medical Center and allows instructors to receive immediate feedback on how well students understand the lecture material. The Veterinary Teaching Hospital has one of the largest caseloads in the country. Outstanding faculty are involved in teaching veterinary students, providing patient treatment and diagnostic services, and conducting veterinary research.

Application Information

Applications available: May

Application deadline: October 1

Application fee: see VMCAS

Residency implications: priority given to Michigan residents. Admission of nonresident and international applicants is limited. Michigan State University has no contractual agreements.

Veterinary Medical College Application Service (VMCAS): required for all applicants.

Prerequisites for Admission

Course requirements and semester hours
  General education
English composition	3
Social and behavioral sciences	6
Humanities	6

  Mathematics and biological and physical sciences
General inorganic chemistry (with laboratory)	3–5
Organic chemistry (with laboratory)	6–8
Biochemistry*	4
General biology (with laboratory)	6–9
College algebra and trigonometry	3–5
College physics (with laboratory)	8

* This should be an upper-division course in general biochemistry.

Required undergraduate GPA: none; the mean cumulative GPA for the last entering class (fall 1999) was 3.63 on a 4.00 scale.

AP credit policy: not available.

Course completion deadline: prerequisite courses must be completed by the end of the summer session prior to matriculation.

Standardized examinations: Medical College Admission Test (MCAT) or the Graduate Record Examination (GRE), general test, is required no later than October. For applicants to the class of 2005, the most recent acceptable MCAT test scores are those of the August 2000 exam. The average MCAT scores for the class entering in 1999 were: verbal 7.00, physical sciences 8.00, and biological sciences 8.00. For applicants to the class of 2005, the most recent acceptable GRE test scores are those of the September 30, 2000 exam. For the class entering in 1999, average GRE scores were: verbal 480, quantitative 667, and analytical 670. The Test of English as a Foreign Language (TOEFL) is required for applicants whose primary language is not English.

Additional requirements and considerations
Extracurricular and/or community service activities
Veterinary-related experience
Evaluations
Veterinarian
Applicant's choice (2)
Academic advisor (required for graduate students)

Summary of Admission Procedure

Timetable
Application deadline: October 1
Date interviews are held: January, February, and March
Date acceptances mailed: early April
School begins: late August

Deposit (to hold place in class): $250.00 for residents; $500.00 for nonresidents.

Deferments: are rare.

Evaluation criteria
The 2-phase admission process consists of an academic review and a non-academic review, including an interview and a pre-interview extemporaneous composition.

1999-2000 admissions summary

	Number of Applicants	Number of New Entrants
Resident	227	85
Nonresident	1,091	18
Total:	1,318	103

Expenses for the 1999-2000 Academic Year

Tuition and fees
Resident $10,788.00
Nonresident $21,900.00

Early Admission Program

The Veterinary Scholars Admission Program has been established by the College of Veterinary Medicine in cooperation with the Honors College at Michigan State. This program provides an admission opportunity for students who wish to complete a bachelor's degree consisting of advanced, intellectually challenging, and scholarly studies in concert with their entry to the four-year professional veterinary medical degree program. Enrollment at MSU and membership in the Honors College are required to be eligible for this option. Further information may be obtained from the Pre-veterinary Advising Center at the address indicated on page 64. For information on Honors College membership, contact: Honors College, 103 Eustace Hall, Michigan State University, East Lansing, MI 48824; telephone (517) 355-2326; or e-mail: honors@pilot.msu.edu

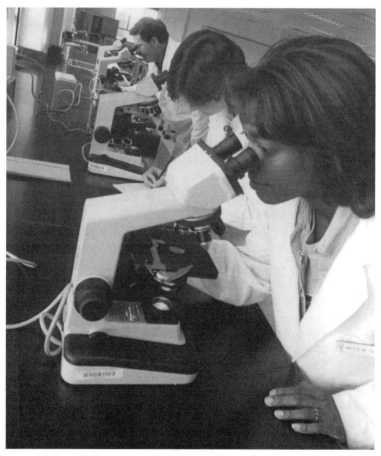

The first- and second-year curriculum for veterinary medical students concentrates on basic science skills. Photo courtesy Oklahoma State University College of Veterinary Medicine.

University of Minnesota

Office of Student Affairs and Admissions
College of Veterinary Medicine
460 Veterinary Teaching Hospital
1365 Gortner Avenue
University of Minnesota
St. Paul MN 55108
Telephone: (612) 624-4747
E-mail: bjork010etc.umn.edu
www.cvm.umn.edu

The University of Minnesota's College of Veterinary Medicine is located on the 540-acre St. Paul campus. Students enjoy a small-campus atmosphere as well as the academic, cultural, social, and recreational opportunities of a major university and large metropolitan area. Cultural life includes world-renowned institutions and a rich local mix of theater, music, and arts organizations. The Twin Cities also house the state capital and the headquarters of many diverse major corporations. Minneapolis and St. Paul consistently rank near the top on quality-of-life and residential satisfaction ratings.

The College of Veterinary Medicine blends cornfields with biotechnology and cow barns with state-of-the-art diagnostic laboratories. The college provides contemporary facilities such as Lewis Hospital for Companion Animals, built in 1983, which is one of the most modern, well-equipped veterinary teaching hospitals in the country, and the Raptor Center, which in 1988 became the world's first facility designed specifically for birds of prey. The educational opportunities extend beyond the campus to include farms throughout Minnesota, the Minnesota Zoo, and even Uruguay and Morocco. Students are given opportunities to learn about the practice of contemporary veterinary medicine through preceptorships, clinical rotations, and first-hand experiences with practitioners.

Application Information

Applications available: May

Application deadline: October 1

Application fee: see VMCAS

Institutional application requirements: $50 application fee

Residency implications: first priority is given to Minnesota residents, minority applicants, and residents of states/provinces with which a reciprocity agreement exists (North Dakota, South Dakota, Manitoba). Residents of other states are encouraged to apply. International applicants are only considered if their preveterinary courses have been completed at a U.S. college or university.

Veterinary Medical College Application Service (VMCAS): required for all applicants.

Prerequisites for Admission

Course requirements and quarter hours

Freshman English, communication	6–9
Mathematics	3–5
Chemistry (with laboratory)	
General inorganic	8–12
General organic*	5–10
Biology (with laboratory)	3–5
Zoology/animal biology (with laboratory)	3–5
Physics (with laboratory)	8–12
Biochemistry	3–5
Genetics	3–5
Microbiology (with laboratory)	3–5
Liberal education	12–18

* Two quarters with one laboratory or one semester with laboratory

A minimum of 4 courses from the following areas of study: anthropology, art, economics, geography, history, humanities, literature (including foreign language literature), music, political science, psychology, public speaking or small group (interpersonal) communication, social science, sociology, theater. No more than 2 courses can be from the same area of study.

Required undergraduate GPA: no minimum required. The class of 2003 had a mean GPA of 3.63 (on a 4.00 scale) for required courses and 3.66 for the last 60 quarter-hour or 45 semester-hour credits of coursework prior to admission.

AP credit policy: must appear on official college transcripts and be equivalent to the appropriate college-level coursework.

Course completion deadline: prerequisite courses must be completed by the end of the spring term (not later than June 15) of the academic year in which application is made.

Standardized examinations: Graduate Record Examination (GRE), general test, is required, and results must be received by January 31. The mean combined score for the 3 tests for the class entering in fall 1999 was 1910.

Summary of Admission Procedure

Timetable

Application deadline: October 1

Date acceptances mailed: mid-April

School begins: early September

Deposit (to hold place in class): $100.00 for Minnesota, Manitoba, South Dakota, and North Dakota residents; $250.00 for nonresidents.

Deferments: can be requested for special circumstances that warrant a 1-year delay in admission.

Evaluation criteria

Objective measures of educational background	70 points
GPA in required courses	20 points
GPA in recent courses	20 points
Test scores	30 points
Subjective measures of personal experience	30 points
Animal/veterinary knowledge, experience, and interest	
Employment record	
Communication skills	
Extracurricular and/or community service activities	
Leadership abilities	
References	
Essay	
Maturity/reliability	

1999-2000 admissions summary

	Number of Applicants	Number of New Entrants
Resident	157	57
Reciprocity*	44	4
Nonresident	876	15
Total:	1,037	76

The figures for new entrants include students taking delayed admission from the previous year.

*For further information, see the listing of contracting states and provinces.

Expenses for the 1999-2000 Academic Year

Tuition and fees

Residents and reciprocity (approximate)	$10,526.00
Nonresidents	$20,006.00

Dual-Degree Programs

Combined DVM-graduate degree programs are available.

Mississippi State University

Office of Student Affairs
College of Veterinary Medicine
P.O. Box 9825
Mississippi State University
Mississippi State MS 39762
Telephone: (601) 325-1129
E-mail: coats@cvm.msstate.edu
www.cvm.msstate.edu

Mississippi State University is located in Starkville (population 20,000). The university has an enrollment of over 15,000. Places of historical interest are prevalent throughout the area. Temperatures are moderate, ranging from the 40s in January to the 90s in July. Air service to the area is 15 minutes away with daily flights that connect with Memphis, Atlanta, and Nashville.

Each class in the College of Veterinary Medicine has 49 students. The curriculum involves 2 primary learning environments: a problem-based learning mode in which students learn basic and clinical sciences through exposure to simulated cases in small group settings, and an experiential mode in which students are rotated through each functional area of the veterinary teaching hospital assisting in primary diagnosis and care. Significant elective opportunities allow students the flexibility to focus study by species, species group, or discipline. A college-wide computer network coupled with a student computer requirement facilitates student communication and access to up-to-date veterinary medical information. Visitors are welcome at the College of Veterinary Medicine and are invited to telephone the Office of Student Affairs. The college suggests calling 2 weeks ahead of the proposed visit so that an appointment may be scheduled.

Application Information

Applications available: July

Application deadline: October 1

Application fee: see VMCAS

Institutional application requirements: $30.00 application fee

Residency implications: Mississippi accepts up to 19 nonresident students.

Veterinary Medical College Application Service (VMCAS): required for all nonresident applicants.

Prerequisites for Admission

Science and math courses must be on the level of those required for preveterinary, predentistry, or science majors and must be completed or updated within 6 calendar years prior to anticipated date of enrollment.

Course requirements and semester hours

Communication	
English composition	6
Oral communication	3
Biological sciences, with laboratories: microbiology, vertebrate zoology, cell biology, genetics	14
Physical sciences, with laboratories: inorganic chemistry, organic chemistry, biochemistry, physics	18
Mathematics	
College algebra, analytic geometry, trigonometry, calculus, finite mathematics, or statistics	6
Nutrition	3–5
Humanities, fine arts, and social/behavioral sciences	15

Required undergraduate GPA: a minimum GPA of 2.80 on a 4.00 scale. The required prerequisite and science GPA is 3.00. The class of 2003 has an average undergraduate GPA of 3.62.

AP credit policy: must appear on official college transcripts and be equivalent to the appropriate college-level coursework.

Course completion deadline: prerequisites must be completed prior to matriculation in late May/early June.

Standardized examinations: Veterinary College Admission Test (VCAT) or Graduate Record Exam (GRE), general test.

Additional requirements and considerations
Evaluation of written application
Confidential evaluations
Interview (by invitation on a competitive basis)

Summary of Admission Procedure

Timetable
Application deadline: October 1
Date interviews are held: late February–early March
Date acceptances mailed: mid-March
School begins: late May–early June

Deposit (to hold place in class): $500.00.

Deferments: requests are considered on an individual basis.

Evaluation criteria	% weight
Grades	50
Test scores	10
Interview; animal/veterinary experience	25
References (3 required, one by a veterinarian)	5
Application (includes essay)	10

1999–2000 admissions summary

		Number of Applicants	Number of New Entrants
Resident		80	30
Nonresident		420	19
	Total:	500	49

Expenses for the 1999/2000 Academic Year

Tuition and fees

Tuition	$6,000.00
Professional Education Fee*	$12,554.00
Activities fee	$1,088.00

* Assessment of the Professional Education Fee is based upon participation in the Mississippi tax system, and state of legal residency is not a factor.

Dual-Degree Programs

Combined DVM-graduate degree programs are available.

University of Missouri

Office of Academic Affairs
College of Veterinary Medicine
W203 Veterinary Medicine Building
University of Missouri-Columbia
Columbia MO 65211
Telephone: (573) 884-6435
E-mail: seayk@missouri.edu
www.missouri.edu

The University of Missouri, with its 23,000 students, is located in Columbia, Missouri. The city of 76,000 is situated 125 miles from St. Louis and Kansas City and about 100 miles north of the Missouri Ozarks. Columbia is a city of 3 colleges, some light industry, major insurance companies, and a number of health-related facilities, including a medical school, and a veterans' hospital, in addition to the veterinary medical college.

The city and campus provide many cultural activities and sporting events. Living conditions are good, and housing is plentiful. Many students elect to live in the country, which is only a short distance from the College of Veterinary Medicine. Hunting for turkey, deer, quail, and other game is available. Fishing throughout the state ranges from farm ponds to large lakes and clear running streams. The climate is generally mild, although some parts of the summer are hot and humid. Winter may have a few days of snow or ice.

Application Information

Applications available: July to mid-October

Application deadline: October 1

Application fee: $50.00

Residency implications: first priority is given to Missouri residents; second priority is given to nonresidents. U.S. citizenship or permanent residency is required.

Veterinary Medical College Application Service (VMCAS): required for nonresident applicants.

Prerequisites for Admission

Course requirements and semester hours

English or communication	6
College algebra or more advanced mathematics	3
Inorganic chemistry	8
Organic chemistry (with laboratory)	5
Physics	5
Biological science	10
Social sciences or humanities	10
Electives	10
Biochemistry	3

Required undergraduate GPA: a cumulative GPA of 2.50 or more on a 4.00 scale is required for Missouri residents. Nonresidents must have a cumulative GPA of 3.00 or more. The most recent entering class had a mean GPA of 3.57 at the time of acceptance.

AP credit policy: not accepted unless documented on University of Missouri transcript.

Course completion deadline: prerequisite courses must be completed by the end of the winter semester or spring quarter of the year of entry.

Standardized examinations: Veterinary College Admission Test (VCAT) is required. Scores must be received by the Admissions Office by February 1. A minimum composite percentile score of 20 is required. The most recent entering class had a mean score of 63.5.

Additional requirements and considerations

Animal/veterinary experience
Recommendations/evaluations (3 required)
    Employer
    Academic advisors/faculty member
    Veterinarians
Extracurricular and/or community service activities
Essays
    Animal experience
    Explanation of choice of veterinary medicine as a profession
Employment history

Summary of Admission Procedure

Timetable

Application deadline: October 1 (nonresidents); November 1 (residents)
Date interviews are held: February–March
Date acceptances mailed: mid-April
School begins: late August

Deposit (to hold place in class): $100.00 for residents; $250.00 for nonresidents.

Deferments: each is considered individually by the admissions committee.

Evaluation criteria
The admission process consists of a file review of all applicants and a personal interview of residents only.

	% weight
Grades	50
Test scores	5
Animal/veterinary experience	15
Interview	10
References	10
Essay	10

1999–2000 admissions summary

		Number of Applicants	Number of New Entrants
Resident		152	54
Nonresident		69	10
	Total:	221	64

Expenses for the 1999-2000 Academic Year

Tuition and fees

Resident	$10,248.00
Nonresident	$19,918.00

Dual-Degree Programs

Combined DVM–graduate degree programs are available.

Early Admission Program

The Pre-veterinary Medicine Scholars Program guarantees acceptance into the professional program upon satisfactory completion of the undergraduate requirements. Eligibility requires a high-school senior or University of Missouri freshman to have a composite ACT score of at least 30, or an equivalent SAT score. Eligible applicants will be interviewed, and a satisfactory score must be achieved to become a Pre-Vet Med Scholar. Selected veterinary medical faculty will be assigned as mentors. Scholars receive priority consideration for part-time employment in the college. Further information may be obtained by contacting the Office of Academic Affairs at the address indicated on page 75.

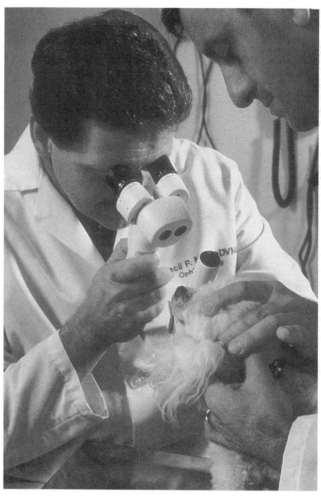

Ophthalmology is one of several specialty areas taught at the University of Missouri's College of Veterinary Medicine. Photo courtesy University of Missouri College of Veterinary Medicine.

North Carolina State University

Student Services Office
College of Veterinary Medicine
4700 Hillsborough Street
North Carolina State University
Raleigh NC 27606
Telephone: (919) 829-6262
E:mail: karen_potter@ncsu.edu
www.cvm.ncsu.edu

The North Carolina State College of Veterinary Medicine is located on a 182-acre site in Raleigh, which has a population of more than 273,000. The sandy shores of North Carolina's beautiful coastline are a short ride to the east, and the Great Smoky Mountains are to the west. The climate includes mild winters and warm summers.

The College of Veterinary Medicine opened in the fall of 1981 and occupies more than 260,000 square feet, including a teaching hospital, classrooms, animal wards, research and teaching laboratories, and an audiovisual area. The college has 120 faculty members and a capacity for 288 veterinary medical students with training for interns, residents, and graduate students.

Application Information

Applications available: May

Application deadline: October 1

Application fee: see VMCAS

Residency implications: priority is given to North Carolina residents. There are approximately 12 nonresident positions.

Veterinary Medical College Application Service (VMCAS): required for all applicants.

Prerequisites for Admission

Course requirements and semester hours

English composition, rhetoric, and reading	6
College calculus	4
Introduction to statistics	3
General physics I, II (with laboratory)	8
General chemistry I (with laboratory)	4
Principles of chemistry (with laboratory)	4
Organic chemistry I, II (with laboratory)	8
General biology (with laboratory)	4
Principles of genetics	4
General microbiology (with laboratory)	4
Biochemistry	3
Animal nutrition	3
Social sciences and the humanities (each)	6

AP credit policy: not available.

Course completion deadline: only 2 courses may be pending completion in the spring semester, and both must be completed (with transcript evidence) by the end of the spring semester prior to matriculation. Pending courses (including correspondence courses) may not be completed in summer sessions.

Standardized examinations: Graduate Record Examination (GRE), general test, is required. The scores must be received by VMCAS by the October 1 application deadline.

Additional requirements and considerations
Animal/veterinary knowledge, experience, motivation, and maturity
Personal statement
Recommendations/evaluations by 3 persons of the applicant's choice (it is encouraged that at least two evaluators be veterinarians unrelated to the applicant)
Extracurricular activities

Summary of Admission Procedure

Timetable
Application deadline: October 1
Date acceptances mailed: third week in March
School begins: August

Deposit (to hold place in class): $250.00.

Deferments: are considered for 1 year only, subject to Admissions Committee approval.

Evaluation criteria
Selection for admission is a 2-phase process:
  Objective score:
    Required course GPA
    Cumulative GPA
    GPA in last 45+ credits attempted
    Test score
  Subjective score:
    Folder review

1999-2000 admissions summary

		Number of Applicants	*Number of New Entrants**
Resident		238	61
Nonresident		907	13
	Total:	1,145	74

* Estimated

Expenses for the 1999-2000 Academic Year

Tuition and fees (estimated)
  Resident $4,000.00
  Nonresident $23,000.00

Dual Degree Programs

Combined DVM-graduate degree programs are available.

Early Admission Program

Two special admissions options are available: (1) for North Carolina residents focusing on swine or poultry medicine in concert with the College of Agriculture and Life Sciences, and (2) for students focusing on laboratory animal medicine in concert with the College of Agriculture at North Carolina A&T State University.

The Ohio State University

Chairperson, Admissions Committee
College of Veterinary Medicine
0004 Veterinary Hospital
601 Tharp Street
The Ohio State University
Columbus OH 43210-1089
Telephone: (614) 292-8831
Fax: (614) 262-6989
E:mail: fenner.2@osu.edu
www.vet.ohio-state.edu/docs/

Ohio State University is located in Columbus, the capital of Ohio. Columbus is a congregation of cities and villages with a sense of history and a friendly atmosphere. The third-ranking center of scientific and technological research and data dissemination in the United States, the city offers fine arts, restaurants, sports, architecture, nature, community festivals, churches, and other areas of interest.

The Ohio State University is one of the nation's leading academic centers, with a sprawling campus straddling the Olentangy River. The campus consists of thousands of acres, hundreds of buildings, more than 15,000 faculty and staff, and more than 54,000 students. The veterinary college is the third-oldest in the United States and is one of the largest veterinary colleges in North America. The patient load is one of the highest in the country, and farmlands can be accessed 10 miles from campus. The faculty members have diverse academic and research activities, and 85 percent of the clinical teaching faculty are board certified. The academic curriculum is a 4-year program that blends some clinical experience into the first 2 years, while the last 2 years are mostly clinical.

Application Information

Applications available: June

Application deadline: October 1

Application fee: see VMCAS

Institutional application requirements: $30.00 application fee

Residency implications: priority is given to Ohio residents. Ohio contracts are with Nevada (1) and West Virginia (5). Ohio will consider qualified nonresident students.

Veterinary Medical College Application Service (VMCAS): required for nonresident applicants.

Prerequisites for Admission

For the humanities and social sciences requirement, students are encouraged to elect the courses required for the bachelor of science curriculum. Courses in communication, journalism, sociology, economics, and animal behavior are strongly recommended.

Students enrolled in the preveterinary medicine curriculum are encouraged to take electives that will provide a well-rounded education in addition to those biological sciences preparatory to the veterinary medical curriculum.

Course requirements and quarter hours

English	5
General chemistry (with laboratory)*	15
Organic chemistry*	6
Biochemistry*	5
Biology*	10
Genetics*	5
Microbiology (with laboratory)*	5
Mathematics (algebra and trigonometry)	5
General physics (with laboratory)	10
Humanities and social sciences	20
Electives	10

* Must have been completed within the 10 years preceding the application deadline.

When applying to the College of Veterinary Medicine, graduate students must have a letter from their advisor releasing them from their graduate program if accepted into the veterinary medicine program.

Required undergraduate GPA: the minimum acceptable GPA for Ohio residents is 2.80; however, students with 3.00 average or above will be given preferential consideration. The minimum acceptable GPA for contract-state residents is 3.00 and for nonresidents is 3.40 (on a 4.00 scale). An undergraduate degree is not a requirement. The Ohio State University calculates a single, comprehensive GPA, which will include grades from all college-level work (both graduate and undergraduate) completed by the applicant.

AP credit policy: not available.

Course completion deadline: all but one prerequisite course must be completed by the end of the fall semester or quarter coinciding with submission of the application. The final remaining prerequisite course must be completed at the end of the following term (spring semester or winter quarter). Failure to satisfactorily complete prerequisites will result in automatic loss of a candidate's seat in the class.

Standardized examinations: Scores from one of the following standardized examinations must be submitted at the time of application:

Graduate Record Examination (GRE): minimum acceptable score 1500 total of all three subtests.

Medical College Admission Test (MCAT): minimum acceptable score 24 total; score O-T on essay portion (new MCAT).

Veterinary College Admission Test (VCAT): minimum acceptable score 50th percentile.

Scores must not be older than five years prior to the application year. The most recent acceptable date for taking the examination is September 30 of the application year.

Additional requirements and considerations

Minimum of 50 hours work with a veterinarian (volunteer or paid)
Academic improvement/difficulty
Personal evaluations
Involvement in community affairs
Communication/interpersonal skills
Initiative/leadership
Attitude/motivation/judgment
Work record/financial responsibility
Social and personal support systems
Comprehensiveness of veterinary medical/animal work experience
Comparative medical experience

Summary of Admission Procedure

Timetable

Application deadline: October 1
Date interviews are held: November–March
Date acceptances mailed: December–March
School begins: late September

Deposit (to hold place in class): $25.00 for residents; $300.00 for contract and nonresident applicants.

Deferments: not considered.

Evaluation criteria

	% weight
Grades	40
Test scores	5
Interview*	55

* Preferred applicants are interviewed and evaluated by members of the Admissions Committee. The academic interview covers subjective areas such as academic improvement versus difficulty, communication/interpersonal skills, involvement in social and community activities, social and personal support systems, work record/financial responsibility, motivation and commitment to veterinary medicine, comprehension of veterinary medicine, knowledge of and/or exposure to animals, and references. Those applicants given the highest overall evaluation are selected for the entering class.

1999–2000 admissions summary

		Number of Applicants	Number of New Entrants
Resident		321	104
Contract*		107	9
Nonresident		584	23
	Total:	1,012	136

Expenses for the 1999-2000 Academic Year

Tuition and fees

Resident	$10,218.00
Nonresident†	$29,613.00

* For further information, see the listing of contracting states and provinces.

† Contract students are assessed the nonresident tuition and fees. The contract state subsidy is subtracted from that tuition, and the student pays the balance due.

Dual-Degree Programs

Combined DVM–graduate degree programs are available.

Oklahoma State University

Admissions Office
College of Veterinary Medicine
Oklahoma State University
Stillwater OK 74078-2003
Telephone: (405) 744-6653
E-mail: vmadmps@okstate.edu
www.okstate.edu

Oklahoma State University is located in Stillwater, which has a population of about 42,000. Stillwater is in north central Oklahoma about 65 miles from Oklahoma City and 69 miles from Tulsa. The campus is exceptionally beautiful, with modified Georgian-style architecture in the new buildings. It encompasses 840 acres and more than 60 major academic buildings.

Three major buildings form the veterinary medicine complex. The oldest, Veterinary Medicine, houses the William E. Brock Memorial Library and Learning Center, as well as new classrooms and laboratories. The Boren Veterinary Medical Teaching Hospital provides the most modern facilities for both academic and clinical instruction. Completing the triad is the Oklahoma Animal Disease Laboratory, which provides both teaching resources and services to Oklahoma agriculture and industry. The College of Veterinary Medicine is fully accredited by the American Veterinary Medical Association. Faculty members in the 3 academic departments share responsibility for the curriculum. These departments are Veterinary Medicine and Surgery; Infectious Diseases and Physiology; and Anatomy, Pathology, and Pharmacology. The latter 2 departments also offer graduate programs for the MS and PhD degrees.

Application Information

Applications available: May

Application deadline: October 1

Application fee: see VMCAS

Residency implications: priority is given to Oklahoma residents. Nonresidents may apply, and Oklahoma State could admit up to 4 contract students from New Jersey and up to 14 first-time nonresident students (including any contract students from Arkansas).

Veterinary Medical College Application Service (VMCAS): required for all applicants.

Prerequisites for Admission

Course requirements and semester hours

English composition	6
English elective	2
General chemistry (with laboratory)	8
Organic chemistry (with laboratory)	8
Biochemistry	3
Physics	8
Mathematics	3
Zoology (with laboratory)	4
Animal nutrition	3
Biological science elective	3
Microbiology (with laboratory)	4
Genetics (laboratory recommended)	3
Humanities or social sciences	6
Electives (science or business)	2

Required undergraduate GPA: a minimum GPA of 2.80 on a 4.00 scale is required in prerequisite courses. The mean cumulative GPA of the 1999 entering class was 3.48.

AP credit policy: not available.

Alternative admissions: in the interest of social justice and cultural diversity, the Oklahoma State Regents for Higher Education permit the college to accept up to 15 percent of a beginning class who do not meet minimum requirements. Limited to Oklahoma residents.

Course completion deadline: prerequisite courses must be completed by the end of the spring semester just prior to matriculation.

Standardized examinations: Graduate Record Examination (GRE), general test and biology subject test, is required. Earliest acceptable test date is June 1996. The class of 2003 had mean scores of 495 verbal, 585 quantitative, 599 analytical, and 508 biology.

Additional requirements and considerations

Evidence of motivation over an extended period of time
Animal/veterinary work experience
Amount of undergraduate education completed

Recommendations/evaluations (3 required)
  Academic advisor, preferred
  Employer
  Veterinarian
Demonstrated leadership and interpersonal skills
All science courses must have been taken within the past 8 years of application (fall 1992)

Summary of Admission Procedure

Timetable
  Application deadline: October 1
  Date interviews held: February
  Date acceptances mailed: March
  School begins: mid- to late August

Deposit (to hold place in class): resident, $100.00; nonresident, $500.00.

Deferments: to complete graduate degree, deferments are considered.

Evaluation criteria
The admission procedure consists of evaluation of both academic and nonacademic criteria. The Admissions Committee considers all factors in the applicant's file, but the following are especially important: academic ability; familiarity with the profession and sincerity of interest; recommendations; test scores; extracurricular activities; character, personality, and general fitness and commitment for a career in veterinary medicine. The committee selects those applicants considered most capable of excelling as veterinary medical students and who possess the greatest potential for success in veterinary medicine.

1999–2000 admissions summary

		Number of Applicants	Number of New Entrants
Resident		120	56
Nonresident		350	18
	Total:	470	74

Expenses for the 1998-99 Academic Year

Tuition and fees
  Resident $7,300.00
  Nonresident $19,100.00

Dual-Degree Programs
Combined DVM–graduate degree programs are available.

Oregon State University

Office of the Dean
College of Veterinary Medicine
Oregon State University
200 Magruder Hall
Corvallis OR 97331-4801
Telephone: (541) 737-2098
Fax: (541) 737-4245
E-mail: cvmproginfo@orst.edu
www.vet.orst.edu

At Oregon State University's College of Veterinary Medicine, students learn the skills to treat and prevent animal diseases through a rigorous course of study taught by a dedicated faculty.

The city of Corvallis, home of OSU, is a modern city of approximately 50,000 that boasts theaters and parks, an art center and shopping malls, and public transportation and bicycle paths to every corner of the community. Life in Corvallis includes lectures, concerts, films, and exhibits through the university. Students can explore the great outdoors just over an hour away by car at the spectacular Oregon coast, the snow-capped Oregon Cascades, and the city of Portland. In the heart of the agriculturally rich Willamette River Valley, Corvallis enjoys colorful and crisp autumns, mild and rainy winters, flowering springs, and warm, dry summers.

Each year, OSU accepts 28 students from Oregon and a total of 8 students from the western regional contract states (Alaska, Arizona, Hawaii, Montana, Nevada, New Mexico, North Dakota, Utah, and Wyoming) and all other states except Washington and Idaho. The first year of professional study is at OSU. Students then transfer to Washington State University in Pullman for the second year and half of the third year of study; then return to Corvallis to complete the remainder of their third year and also their fourth and final year of professional instruction. The small class size and the shared approach to veterinary medical education, unique in the United States, helps to provide the students with an excellent veterinary education and the opportunity to interact with faculty and students of 2 prestigious veterinary colleges.

Application Information

Applications available: May

Application deadline: November 1

Application fee: see VMCAS

Residency implications: Oregon residents and WICHE-sponsored students are eligible for resident fees. A limited number of students are accepted as nonresidents.

Veterinary Medical College Application Service (VMCAS): required for all applicants.

Prerequisites for Admission

Course requirements and quarter hours

Chemistry	A sequence of inorganic chemistry with laboratories; organic chemistry sufficient to meet requirements for upper-division biochemistry course or course sequence; and at least one upper-division biochemistry course
Mathematics	Sufficient to meet the prerequisite for physics and inorganic chemistry (at least college-level algebra)
Physics	2 quarters or 1 semester of college-level physics for science majors
Zoology or biology	1 year sequence
Genetics	1 quarter or semester
Biological sciences	A minimum of at least 6 additional quarter hours or 4 semester hours of upper-division biological science courses, with at least one laboratory (physiology, cell physiology, cell biology, microbiology, or additional biochemistry)

Total minimum number of credits required: 107 quarter credits; 72 semester credits.

Required undergraduate GPA: overall GPA must be at least 3.00 or the last 2 years must be at least 3.00. The mean overall GPA for the class entering in fall of 1999 was 3.46.

AP credit policy: must appear on official college transcripts and be equivalent to the appropriate college-level coursework.

Course completion deadline: prerequisite courses must be completed by June 15 prior to entry.

Standardized examinations: Graduate Record Examination (GRE), general test, is required. The most recent acceptable test date for applicants to the class of 2005 is November 30, 2000. The mean score of the 1999 entering class was at the 59.52 percentile.

Additional requirements and considerations:

Animal/veterinary work experience: applicants must have some veterinary medical exposure and animal work experience by November 1 of the year of application to be considered for admission. Working with veterinarians is the most common approach to fulfilling this requirement. Some credit will be given for animal experience such as breeding, rearing, feeding, and showing various species of animals, including companion animals, livestock, laboratory animals, zoo animals, or wildlife. Experience in veterinary clinics and hospitals and in research laboratories is highly encouraged.

Recommendations (3 required, one by a veterinarian)

Extracurricular and/or community service activities desirable

Summary of Admission Procedure

Timetable

Application deadline: November 1

Date interviews are held: late February to early March

Date acceptances mailed: mid-March

School begins: late September

Deposit (to hold place in class): $50.00

Deferments: are rare.

Evaluation criteria

The admission procedure consists of 2 parts: a file review and a personal interview of applicants considered to be competitive. (Interviews for non-residents and WICHE students may not be required.)

	% weight
Grades	36
Test scores	7
Animal/veterinary experience	15
Interview	24
References, personal development	11
Academic index: quality and quantity of course load, work commitments, etc.	7

(Additional points may be awarded in a "diversity/adversity" category.)

1999–2000 admissions summary

	Number of Applicants	Number of New Entrants
Resident	114	28
Contract (WICHE)*	186	1
Nonresident	685	7
Total:	985	36

Expenses for the 1999–2000 Academic Year

Tuition and fees

Resident (approximate)	$10,275.00
Nonresident	
Contract*	$10,275.00
Other nonresident (approximate)	$20,058.00

* For further information, see the listing of contracting states and provinces.

Dual-Degree Programs

Combined DVM-graduate degree programs are available.

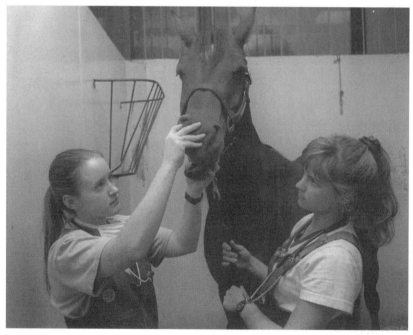

Students examine the mucous membranes of an equine patient at the College of Veterinary Medicine at Oregon State University. Photo courtesy Oregon State University College of Veterinary Medicine.

University of Pennsylvania

Admissions Office
School of Veterinary Medicine
3800 Spruce Street
University of Pennsylvania
Philadelphia PA 19104-6044
Telephone: (215) 898-5434
E-mail: admissions@vet.upenn.edu
www.vet.upenn.edu

The University of Pennsylvania is located in West Philadelphia. Philadelphia is a city with a strong cultural heritage. Independence National Park includes 1 square mile of historic Philadelphia next to the Delaware River. Included are Independence Hall, the Liberty Bell, and many fine examples of colonial architecture. Philadelphia also offers theaters, museums, sports, and outdoor recreation. The Philadelphia Zoo, first in the nation, houses more than 1,600 mammals, birds, reptiles, and amphibians. The School of Veterinary Medicine enjoys a close relationship with the zoo.

The School of Veterinary Medicine was founded in 1884 and includes a hospital for small animals, classrooms, and research facilities in the city. The large-animal hospital and research facilities are located at the New Bolton Center, an 800-acre farm 40 miles west of Philadelphia. The first 2 years are spent on the main campus. Part of the third year may be spent at the New Bolton Center, and the fourth year is spent in rotation and on electives at varying campus locations. Off-campus electives are frequently permitted.

Application Information

Applications available: May

Application deadline: October 1

Application fee: see VMCAS

Residency implications: priority is given to Pennsylvania residents. Contract arrangements are with New Jersey. The number of nonresident places is usually 45–50, including international applicants.

Veterinary Medical College Application Service (VMCAS): required for all applicants.

Prerequisites for Admission

At least 3 English credits must be in composition; biology courses must provide background in genetics. Organic chemistry must cover aliphatic and aromatic compounds to fulfill the requirement.

Course requirements and semester hours

English (including 1 writing course)	6
Physics (with laboratory)	8
Chemistry (with at least 1 laboratory)	
General	8
Organic	4
Biology or zoology (3 courses)	9
Social sciences or humanities	6
Calculus	3
Electives	46

(Although not required, biochemistry is strongly recommended.)

Required undergraduate GPA: no specific GPA. Applicants are evaluated comparatively and should have at least a GPA of 3.30 to be competitive. The mean cumulative GPA of the class admitted in 1999 was 3.50.

AP credit policy: not available.

Course completion deadline: prerequisite courses must be completed by the end of the summer term of the year in which admission is sought.

Standardized examinations: Graduate Record Examination (GRE), general test, is required. Scores should be received no later than December 1. The class admitted in 1999 had an average of 560 on the verbal subtest and 670 on the quantitative subtest.

Additional requirements and considerations

   Animal/veterinary work experience: experience working with animals, direct veterinary work, or research experience is desired. No minimum time limit. Experience should be sufficient to convince the admissions committee of motivation, interest, and understanding.

   Recommendations/evaluations: 3 required, one from an academic science source; and one from a veterinarian. The third is the choice of the applicant.

   Extracurricular/community service activities: additional activities in this category can provide information important to the admissions committee.

   Leadership: evidence of leadership abilities is desirable.

Summary of Admission Procedure

Timetable
>   Application deadline: October 1
>   Date interviews are held: Fridays from late January until completion
>   Date acceptances mailed: within 14 days after interview
>   School begins: early September

Deposit (to hold place in class): $500.00.

Deferments: are considered on an individual basis.

Evaluation criteria
The University of Pennsylvania accepts about 40 percent of each class without interview. The remaining seats are filled through a 2-part admission procedure, which includes a file review and personal interviews.

>   Grades
>   Test scores
>   Animal/veterinary experience
>   Interview
>   References
>   Essay
>   English skills (TOEFL)

File review: files are reviewed in January by pairs of members of the admissions committee (including an alumni member), and decisions are made on whether or not to offer an interview.

Personal interviews: interviews are held on Fridays from late January until the class is filled. The number of interviews granted equals 2 to 3 times the number of seats available.

Two personal interviews are conducted: a formal interview with 2 faculty members (including an alumni member) of the committee, and an informal interview with student committee members. Although students do not vote on acceptance, they have a significant part in the meeting following interviews.

1999–2000 admissions summary

	Number of Applicants	Number of New Entrants
Resident	245	62
Nonresident*	1,132	47
Total:	1,377	109[†]

*   For further information, see listing of contracting states and provinces.
†   Includes 2 international students

95

Expenses for the 1999-2000 Academic Year

Tuition and fees

Resident	$23,570.00
Nonresident	
Contract*	$23,570.00
Other nonresident	$29,238.00

* For further information, see listing of contracting states and provinces.

Dual-Degree Programs

Combined DVM-graduate degree programs are available.

Purdue University

Student Services Office
School of Veterinary Medicine
1240 Lynn Hall
Purdue University
West Lafayette IN 47907-1240
Telephone: (765) 494-7893 or (800) 213-2859 (long distance)
E-mail: admissions@vet.purdue.edu
www.vet.purdue.edu

Purdue University is located in one of the largest metropolitan centers in northwestern Indiana. Greater Lafayette occupies a site on the Wabash River 65 miles northwest of Indianapolis and 126 miles southeast of Chicago. The combined population of the twin cities, Lafayette and West Lafayette, exceeds 64,000. The community offers an art museum, historical museum, 1,600 acres of public parks, and more than 60 churches of all major denominations.

Purdue ranks among the 25 largest colleges and universities in the nation. Students represent all 50 states and many foreign countries. Diversity and opportunity are goals that the School of Veterinary Medicine maintains in the selection of each year's entering class. The School of Veterinary Medicine has assumed a leading position nationally and internationally in veterinary education. To better prepare individuals for veterinary medical careers in the twenty-first century, new and innovative strategies are being implemented into the curriculum.

Application Information

Applications available: May

Application deadline: October 1

Application fee: see VMCAS

Residency implications: priority is given to Indiana residents. Approximately one-third of the class will be nonresident students in a total class of 60. Applicants from all states will be considered. Purdue has no contract positions. International applicants will be considered provided both the academic and financial criteria can be met.

Veterinary Medical College Application Service (VMCAS): required for all applicants.

Prerequisites for Admission

The course requirements outlined below are considered the bare minimum prerequisite courses to be completed. No less than a grade of C must be received in each required course in order to be considered eligible for admission.

In the electives category, humanities include languages, cognitive sciences, and social sciences; business writing and macroeconomics courses are highly recommended. Other courses that are highly recommended include computer, basic and comparative nutrition, and general animal science courses.

Course requirements and semester hours

English composition	6
Speech (public speaking)	3
Biology (with laboratory) (diversity, development, cell structure)	8–13
Chemistry, general (with laboratory)	8–10
Chemistry, organic (with laboratory) or chemistry, organic (with laboratory) (1 semester) and quantitative analysis (1 semester)	8–9
Biochemistry	3–6
Calculus	6–10
Physics (with laboratory)	8
Genetics (with laboratory)	4
Statistics	3
Humanities	9

Required undergraduate GPA: the mean cumulative GPA of the 1999 entering class was 3.59 on a 4.00 scale. The minimum overall GPA required for consideration is 2.50 on a 4.00 scale.

AP credit policy: must appear on official college transcripts and be equivalent to the appropriate college-level coursework.

Course completion deadline: minimum prerequisite courses must be completed by the end of the spring term prior to matriculation.

Standardized examinations: Graduate Record Examination (GRE), general and Writing Assessment tests, is required. Test scores must be received no later than December 1 of the year of application.

Additional requirements and considerations
  Animal/veterinary experience
  Amount of college education
  Recommendations/evaluations (3 required)
    Academic advisor/faculty member
    Employer
    Veterinarian
  Essay
  Employment record
  Extracurricular college experience

Summary of Admission Procedure

Timetable
  Application deadline: October 1
  Date interviews are held: February
  Date acceptances mailed: March
  School begins: late August

Deposit (to hold place in class): $250.00 for residents; $1,000.00 for nonresidents.

Deferments: request for deferments will be considered on a case-by-case basis.

Evaluation criteria
The admission process consists of:
    A preliminary review based upon grade point indices, test scores, and
      prerequisite course completion
    An in-depth review of selected applicants
    A personal interview by invitation

	% weight
Grades, test scores, overall academic performance	50
Animal, veterinary, and general work experiences, extracurricular activities, essay, overall presentation of application materials, references, and interview	50

1999-2000 admissions summary

	Number of Applicants	Number of New Entrants
Resident	118	43
Nonresident	813	25
International	14	0
Total:	945	68

Expenses for the 1999-2000 Academic Year (estimated)

Tuition and fees
Resident	$8,760.00
Nonresident	$21,120.00

Dual-Degree Programs

Combined DVM-graduate degree programs are available.

Early Admission Program

The Veterinary Scholars Program provides an opportunity for early admission into the professional program by accepting high-school seniors who

1. ranked in the top 10 percent of their graduating class;
2. have attained a combined SAT score equal to or greater than 1300 or composite ACT score equal to or greater than 28;
3. were admitted to Purdue University in animal sciences, biochemistry, or biological sciences programs; and
4. demonstrate a background of work experience with animals and veterinarians.

Students admitted to the program must complete all preveterinary prerequisite coursework, obtain a bachelor's degree with stipulated grade point averages for each year of undergraduate study, and submit scores from the GRE (Graduate Record Exam), general test, and the GRE Writing Assessment test during their senior year.

University of Tennessee

Office of the Associate Dean
College of Veterinary Medicine
P.O. Box 1071
University of Tennessee
Knoxville TN 37901-1071
Telephone: (865) 974-7263
E-mail: jbrace@utk.edu
www.vet.utk.edu

The University of Tennessee's College of Veterinary Medicine is located in Knoxville, a city of 169,000 situated in the Appalachian foothills of east central Tennessee. Only 45 minutes from the Great Smoky Mountains National Park and 3 hours from both Nashville and Atlanta, Knoxville offers recreational and cultural opportunities, including a symphony orchestra, an opera company, and several fine theaters. The climate in Knoxville is moderate with distinct seasons.

The 417-acre Knoxville campus of the University of Tennessee has about 20,259 undergraduate and 5,249 graduate students. The modern Clyde M. York Veterinary Medicine Building, housing the teaching and research facilities, Veterinary Teaching Hospital, and Agriculture-Veterinary Medicine Library, faces the Tennessee River on the university's Agricultural Campus.

The curriculum of the College of Veterinary Medicine is a 9-semester, 4-year program. Development of a strong basic science education is emphasized in the first year. The second and third years emphasize the study of diseases, their causes, diagnosis, treatment, and prevention. Innovative features of this curriculum include 8 weeks of student-centered small-group applied-learning exercises in semesters 1-6; 3 weeks of dedicated clinical experiences in the veterinary teaching hospital in semesters 3-5; and elective course opportunities in semesters 4-6 that allow students to focus on specific educational/career goals. In the fourth year, students participate exclusively in clinical rotations in the Veterinary Teaching Hospital and required off-campus externships. The college has unique programs in zoo and exotic animal medicine and surgery, cancer diagnosis and therapy, endoscopy, and laser surgery.

Application Information

Applications available: May

Application deadline: November 1

Application fee: see VMCAS

Institutional application requirements: $35 application fee

Residency implications: priority is given to Tennessee residents. Tennessee has no contractual agreements and does accept nonresident applications.

Veterinary Medical College Application Service (VMCAS): required for all applicants.

Prerequisites for Admission

Course requirements and semester hours

General inorganic chemistry (with laboratory)	8
Organic chemistry (with laboratory)	8
General biology/zoology (with laboratory)	8
Cellular biology*	3
Genetics	3
Biochemistry (exclusive of laboratory)†	4
Physics (with laboratory)	8
English composition	6
Social sciences/humanities	18

* Applicants are strongly encouraged to complete additional biological science courses, especially comparative anatomy, mammalian physiology, and microbiology with laboratory.

† This should be a complete upper-division course in general cellular and comparative biochemistry. Half of a 2-semester sequence will not satisfy this requirement.

AP credit policy: must appear on official college transcripts and be equivalent to the appropriate college-level coursework.

Required undergraduate GPA: for nonresident applicants, the minimum acceptable cumulative GPA is 3.20 on a 4.00 scale. At time of acceptance, the mean GPA of the class entering in fall of 1999 was 3.56.

Course completion deadline: prerequisite courses must be completed with a grade of C or better by the end of the spring term prior to entry.

Standardized examinations: Veterinary College Admission Test (VCAT) is required. For applicants planning to matriculate in August 2001, the oldest acceptable VCAT scores are from the October 1998 test date.

Additional requirements and considerations
  Animal/veterinary work experience
  Recommendations/evaluations
  Extracurricular and/or community service activities
  Leadership skills
  Autobiographical essay (personal statement)

Summary of Admission Procedure

Timetable
  Application deadline: November 1
  Date interviews are held: mid- to late March
  Date acceptances mailed: no later than April 1
  Applicant's response date: April 15
  School begins: late August

Deposit (to hold place in class): none required.

Deferments: are considered on a case-by-case basis.

Evaluation criteria
The University of Tennessee's admission procedure consists of an initial file review followed by an interview of selected applicants.

  Grades
  Test scores   } Initial academic file review.
  Animal/veterinary experience
  Interview
  References (3 required)
  Essay
(Evaluation is not percentage based.)

1999–2000 admissions summary

	Number of Applicants	Number of New Entrants
Resident	156	65
Nonresident	315	0
Total:	471	65

Expenses for the 1999–2000 Academic Year

Tuition and fees
  Resident $6,160.00
  Nonresident $15,738.00

Texas A & M University

Office of the Dean
College of Veterinary Medicine
Texas A & M University
College Station TX 77843-4461
Telephone: (409) 845-5038
www.cvm.tamu.edu

The university is located adjacent to the cities of Bryan and College Station. The 2 cities have a combined population of about 100,000. The student population at Texas A & M is more than 40,000. The College of Veterinary Medicine is one of the 10 original veterinary teaching institutions that existed in the United States prior to World War II.

Application Information

Applications available: May

Application deadline: October 1

Application fee: see VMCAS

Residency implications: Texas has no contractual agreements with other states. Applicants from other states who have outstanding credentials will be considered. Successful candidates who are awarded competitive university-based scholarships may attend at resident tuition rate.

Veterinary Medical College Application Service (VMCAS): required for all applicants.

Prerequisites for Admission

The minimum number of college or university credits required for admission into the professional curriculum is 64 semester hours. Applicants must have completed or have in progress approximately 48 credit hours at the time of application. Because there is no specific degree plan associated with preveterinary education, students are encouraged to pursue a degree plan that meets individual interests. Students are strongly encouraged to choose courses with the assistance of a knowledgeable counselor at the undergraduate institution or through contact with an academic advisor at the College of Veterinary Medicine, Texas A & M University, telephone: (800) 874-9591.

Course requirements and semester hours

Life sciences

General biology (with laboratory)   4
  Survey of contemporary biology that covers the
  chemical basis of life, structure and biology of the cell,
  molecular biology, and genetics

General microbiology (with laboratory)   4
  Basic microbiology; comparative morphology,
  taxonomy, pathogenesis, ecology, variation, and
  physiology of microorganisms

Genetics   3
  Basic concepts of mammalian genetics

Animal nutrition or feeds and feeding   3
  Emphasis on basic principles of animal nutrition;
  nutritional roles of carbohydrates, proteins, lipids,
  minerals, vitamins, and water; emphasis on digestion,
  absorption, metabolism, and excretion of the nutrients
  and their metabolites

Chemical-physical sciences and mathematics

Inorganic chemistry (with laboratory)   8
  Basic concepts of modern inorganic chemistry

Organic chemistry (with laboratory)   4
  Basic concepts of modern organic chemistry

Biochemistry   3
  An introduction to the chemistry and metabolism of
  biologically important molecules, the biochemical basis
  of life processes, and cellular metabolism and regulation

Calculus/statistics   3

Physics (with laboratory)   8
  Fundamentals of mechanics, heat, sound, electricity, and light

Nonscience

Composition and rhetoric   3
Literature   3
Speech communication   3
Technical writing   3

Additional credits

In addition to the 52 credit hours recommended above, an applicant must complete a minimum of 12 additional credits. Applicants should keep in mind their degree program, the core curriculum requirements for a baccalaureate degree at Texas A & M University, and their personal career goals in making these choices. Applicants are strongly encouraged to make these choices with a qualified counselor at their institution.

Required undergraduate GPA: the minimum overall GPA required is 2.90 on a 4.00 scale or 3.10 for the last 45 semester credits. The mean of the most recent entering class was 3.60.

AP credit policy: not available.

Course completion deadline: required courses must be completed by the end of the spring term prior to entry.

Standardized examinations: Graduate Record Examination (GRE), general test, is required. Standardized test scores must be 5 years old or less. The class entering in 1999 averaged 1871 (combined verbal, quantitative, and analytical subtests) on the GRE.

Additional requirements and considerations

Evaluations
Animal/veterinary work experience

Knowledge and experience in working with animals is crucial to becoming a successful veterinarian. While the professional curriculum is almost totally devoted to the understanding of animals, animal contact, experience, and handling should also be major considerations in the preveterinary training period. Applicants are expected to be familiar with animal systems and behavior. For those interested in farm animal veterinary medicine, general agriculture knowledge should also be a major consideration. To obtain this experience, applicants should either register for coursework based on their background, interests, and needs, or involve themselves in practical animal operations in the private sector. If designated courses in the animal sciences are not available at the applicant's institution, demonstrable experience with animals is acceptable. Formal training in animal systems and animal behavior is highly desirable and encouraged if available at the applicant's institution.

Summary of Admission Procedure

Timetable
    Application deadline: October 1
    Date interviews are held: before February 15
    Date acceptances mailed: March
    School begins: late August

Deposit (to hold place in class): none required.

Deferments: requests for deferments will be considered on a case-by-case basis.

Evaluation criteria
    Academic performance
    Test scores
    Interview
    Personal statement
    Personal evaluations (3 evaluations are required)
    Semester course load and postacademic challenge
    Leadership and experience

1999–2000 admissions summary

		Number of Applicants	Number of New Entrants
Resident		394	121
Nonresident		562	7
	Total:	956	128

Expenses for the 1999–2000 Academic Year

Tuition and fees
Resident	$8,035.00
Nonresident	$18,835.00

Tufts University

Office of Admissions
School of Veterinary Medicine
200 Westboro Road
Tufts University
North Grafton MA 01536
Telephone: (508) 839-7920
E-mail: vetadmissions@infonet.tufts.edu
www.tufts.edu/vet/

Tufts University is located near Boston, where sports and cultural activities abound. The School of Veterinary Medicine provides an exciting biomedical environment for the study of modern veterinary medicine. Signature programs include wildlife medicine, equine sports medicine, international veterinary medicine, biotechnology and veterinary medicine, and the study of issues related to ethical dimensions of veterinary medicine, including animal welfare.

Hands-on learning begins in the first year with a course on clinical skills and animal behavior and continues throughout the next 3 years. Many opportunities exist outside of formal courses for hands-on work in hospitals and research laboratories. The Hospital for Large Animals, Foster Hospital for Small Animals, the Ambulatory Clinic, and the Wildlife Clinic provide a rich mixture of horses, cats, dogs, cattle, sheep, goats, and native wildlife.

Application Information

Applications available: July

Application deadline: December 1

Application fee: $60.00 on line; $75.00 hard copy

Residency implications: Massachusetts residents make up about half of each class. All others considered for the remaining spaces. Tufts contracts with Maine (1), New Hampshire (1-2), and New Jersey (6).

Veterinary Medical College Application Service (VMCAS): no participation.

Prerequisites for Admission

Course requirements and semesters

Biology (with laboratory)	2
Inorganic chemistry (with laboratory)	2
Organic chemistry (with laboratory)	2
Physics	2
Mathematics	2
Genetics, unless included in biology	1
Biochemistry	1
English composition	2
Social and behavioral sciences	2
Humanities and fine arts	2

Required undergraduate GPA: no minimum GPA required. The average GPA for the class admitted in 1999 was 3.47.

AP credit policy: must appear on official college transcripts and be equivalent to the appropriate college-level coursework.

Course completion deadline: prerequisite courses must be completed by the time of matriculation into the DVM program.

Standardized examinations: Graduate Record Examination (GRE), general test, is required. The most recent acceptable test date for applicants to the class of 2005 is November 2000. GRE scores are valid for 5 years; the exam must have been taken during or after 1996. Average GRE scores for the class of 2003 were verbal 600, quantitative 680, and analytical 700.

Additional requirements and considerations
Animal/veterinary/biomedical research experience
Recommendations/evaluations (3 required)
advisor/faculty members
veterinarian/research scientist/project leader
Essays
Interview

Summary of Admission Procedure

Timetable
Application deadline: December 1
Date interviews are held: February
Date acceptances mailed: March
School begins: late August

Deposit (to hold place in class): $500.00.

Deferments: requests for deferment are handled on a case-by-case basis.

Evaluation criteria
Tufts' admission procedure consists of a review of the application and an interview of selected applicants.

1999–2000 admissions summary

	Number of Applicants	Number of New Entrants
Total:	768	80

Expenses for the 1999–2000 Academic Year

Tuition and fees

Resident	$23,364.00
Contract*	$15,038.00
Nonresident	$27,038.00

* For further information, see the listing of contracting states and provinces.

Dual-Degree Program

Combined DVM–graduate degree programs are available.

Tuskegee University

School of Veterinary Medicine, Nursing, and Allied Health
Tuskegee University
Tuskegee AL 36088
Telephone: (334) 727-8460

Tuskegee University School of Veterinary Medicine is located in Tuskegee, Alabama, a city of about 25,000. Tuskegee is located about 40 miles east of Montgomery and 40 miles west of Columbus, Georgia. Summers are hot and humid, and winters are moderate. Numerous lakes, parks, recreational facilities, and other educational institutions are located nearby.

The university was founded by Booker T. Washington in 1881, and the veterinary school was established in 1945. Seventy percent of black veterinarians in the United States received their professional training at Tuskegee. A large portion of the campus has been declared a historical site by the National Park Service.

Application Information

Applications available: July

Application deadline: First Monday in December

Application fee: $25.00

Residency implications: applications are accepted nationwide, with a minimum number of contract spaces for Kentucky (2), New Jersey (2), South Carolina (4), and West Virginia (2).

Veterinary Medical College Application Service (VMCAS): no participation.

Prerequisites for Admission

Course requirements and semester hours

English composition/communications	6
Mathematics (algebra and trigonometry)	6
Chemistry (minimum)	
Organic chemistry (with laboratory)	4
Biochemistry (with laboratory)	4
Physics* (with laboratory)	8
Biological science	
Advanced biology**	9
Free electives	8
(advanced biological science—optional)	
Animal science	9
(includes poultry and animal nutrition)	
Social science and humanities	6
Electives—liberal arts	6

* One academic year

** Advanced biology courses, e.g., zoology, microbiology, genetics, anatomy, physiology, and histology

Required undergraduate GPA: the requirement is 2.70 on a 4.00 scale.

AP credit policy: not available.

Course completion deadline: prerequisite courses must be completed by the end of the spring semester of the year of application.

Standardized examinations: Veterinary College Admission Test (VCAT), Medical College Admission Test (MCAT), or Graduate Record Examination (GRE), any of which must be taken within 3 years of application, is required.

Summary of Admission Procedure

Timetable

 Application deadline: First Monday in December
 Date interviews are held: February–March
 Date acceptances mailed: April 15
 School begins: late August

Deposit (to hold place in class): $275.00.

Deferments: one-year deferments are offered upon written request.

Evaluation criteria

The following items are taken into consideration: academic record, academic trends, letters of recommendation, work experience, and test scores.

	% weight
Grades	50
Test scores	5
Animal/veterinary experience	2
Interview	20
References	2
Essay	1

1999-2000 admissions summary

		Number of Applicants	*Number of New Entrants*
Resident		35	7
Contract*		99	23
Nonresident		129	31
	Total:	263	61

Expenses for the 1999-2000 Academic Year

Tuition and fees $12,000.00

* For further information, see the listing of contracting states and provinces.

Dual-Degree Programs

Combined DVM-graduate degree programs are available.

Virginia Polytechnic Institute and State University

Admissions Coordinator
Virginia-Maryland Regional College of Veterinary Medicine
Virginia Polytechnic Institute and State University
Blacksburg VA 24061
Telephone: (540) 231-4699
Fax: (540) 231-9290
E-mail: dvmadmit@vt.edu
www.vetmed.vt.edu

The Virginia-Maryland Regional College of Veterinary Medicine is situated on 3 distinct campuses. The main campus is at Virginia Tech in Blacksburg, Virginia, a community with a population of about 40,000 situated on a high plateau in southwestern Virginia between the Blue Ridge and Allegheny Mountains. Its residents enjoy a wide range of educational, social, recreational, and cultural opportunities. In addition to the Blacksburg campus, the Equine Medical Center campus is in Leesburg, Virginia, and the University of Maryland is at College Park. The college received full accreditation in 1993 from the American Veterinary Medical Association.

In recognition of a need for veterinarians trained in both basic and clinical sciences, the college offers students the opportunity to participate in graduate studies and receive appropriate advanced training to conduct research in basic or clinical disciplines. Nearly 25 percent of the nation's veterinarians work in areas other than private practice, such as government and corporate veterinary medicine. Through the assistance of a grant from the Pew Charitable Trusts, the college has established the Center for Government and Corporate Veterinary Medicine, which is a national resource for training veterinarians for the wide variety of careers in this area of the profession.

Application Information

Applications available: May

Application deadline: October 1

Application fee: see VMCAS

Residency implications: 50 positions are reserved for Virginia residents, and 30 positions for Maryland residents. Virginia contracts with Delaware and offers up to 3 positions for Delaware residents; the remaining positions (7–10) may be filled by nonresidents.

Veterinary Medical College Application Service (VMCAS): required for all applicants.

Prerequisites for Admission

Course requirements and semester hours

Biological sciences (with laboratories)	8
Organic chemistry (with laboratories)	8
Physics (with laboratories)	8
Biochemistry	3
English (composition, 3 credit hours)	6
Humanities/social science	6
Mathematics (algebra, geometry, trigonometry, calculus)	6

Students must earn a C– or better in all required courses.

Science courses taken 7 or more years ago may be repeated or substituted with higher-level courses with the written consent of the admissions committee.

Required undergraduate GPA: to be considered for admission, applicants must have a cumulative GPA of at least 2.80 on a 4.00 scale upon completion of a minimum of 2 academic years of full-time study (60 semester/90 quarter hours) at an accredited college or university. Alternatively, a 3.30 GPA in the last 2 years (60 semester hours) will qualify a student who does not have a 2.80 GPA overall. All courses taken during this 2-year period must be junior or senior level. The mean GPA of those accepted into the class of 2003 was 3.50.

AP credit policy: not available.

Course completion deadline: required courses must be completed by the end of the spring term of the year in which matriculation occurs.

Standardized examinations: Graduate Record Examination (GRE) is required. For the class of 2003, the mean score on the aptitude portion (verbal, quantitative, analytical) was 1850. The oldest acceptable scores must be within 5 years of the application deadline.

Additional requirements and considerations

Maturity and a broad cultural perspective

Motivation and dedication to a career in veterinary medicine

Evidence of potential, and appreciation of the career opportunities for veterinarians, as indicated by:

1. Clinical veterinary experience (private practice)

2. Animal experience in addition to time spent working with a veterinarian
3. Veterinary experience outside of private clinical practice, such as research, industrial, government, and corporate settings
4. Extramural activities, achievements, honors
5. Communication skills
6. References

Summary of Admission Procedure

Timetable

Application deadline: October 1
Date interviews are held: late February/early March
Date acceptances mailed: early March
School begins: mid-August

Deposit (to hold place in class): $450.00 for Maryland and Virginia residents; $1,000.00 for nonresidents.

Deferments: case-by-case basis if a candidate has extenuating circumstances beyond his or her control.

Evaluation criteria

The Virginia-Maryland Regional College of Veterinary Medicine has a 3-part admission procedure, comprised of an initial screening of applicants by the Admissions and Standards Committee with input from the college faculty, an interview of selected applicants, and a final review of the dossiers of all interviewees by the Admissions and Standards Committee.

	% weight
Academics	50
Cumulative GPA, required science GPA, last 45 semester-hour GPA, GRE aptitude	
Background	25
Related animal experience; veterinary experience; research, industrial, and commercial experience; activities, achievements, and awards; narrative and personal references	
Interviews	25

1999-2000 admissions summary

		Number of Applicants	*Number of New Entrants*
Resident			
Maryland		138	30
Virginia		145	50
Contract*		15	3
Nonresident		<u>696</u>	<u>7</u>
	Total:	994	90

Expenses for the 1998-99 Academic Year

Tuition and fees
Resident	$8,912.00
Nonresident	$22,136.00

Dual-Degree Programs

Combined DVM-graduate degree programs are available.

Washington State University

Office of Student Services
College of Veterinary Medicine
Washington State University
Pullman WA 99164-7012
Telephone: (509) 335-1532

Washington State University, which has an enrollment of 20,000, is located in southeastern Washington in the town of Pullman. This small community is surrounded by farmland yet is close to the mountains of Idaho. The area offers excellent summer and winter recreation.

The College of Veterinary Medicine at WSU was founded in 1899 and is one of the 5 oldest colleges of veterinary medicine in the country. Washington, Oregon, and Idaho (WOI) have developed a regional program in veterinary medical education that also serves Alaska, Arizona, Hawaii, Montana, Nevada, New Mexico, North Dakota, Utah, and Wyoming through the Western Interstate Commission for Higher Education (WICHE) Compact.

The DVM degree is awarded by Washington State University and Oregon State University. The University of Idaho is a full partner in the program, but Idaho students receive their DVM degrees from Washington.

Application Information

Applications available: May

Application deadline: October 1

Application fee: see VMCAS

Institutional application requirements: $30 application fee

Residency implications: priority is given to Washington and Idaho residents. WOI contracts with WICHE states (Alaska, Arizona, Hawaii, Montana, Nevada, New Mexico, North Dakota, Utah, Wyoming) for 16 places. Washington accepts a few (approximately 5) nonresidents each year from states other than contracts listed above.

Veterinary Medical College Application Service (VMCAS): required for all applicants.

Prerequisites for Admission

Course requirements

Chemistry	A sequence of inorganic and organic courses with laboratories and one upper-division biochemistry course
Mathematics	Sufficient to meet the prerequisites for inorganic chemistry and physics
Physics	1 semester or equivalent of college-level physics for science majors
Zoology or biology	1-year sequence
Genetics	1 semester or equivalent

Total minimum number of credits required is 60 semester hours or 90 quarter hours.

Required undergraduate GPA: none; a minimum overall GPA of 3.20 (or 3.30 for the last 45 semester credit hours) on a 4.00 scale is recommended. The class of 2003 had a mean overall GPA of 3.67 at the time of acceptance.

AP credit policy: must appear on official college transcripts and be equivalent to the appropriate college-level coursework.

Course completion deadline: prerequisite courses must be completed by June 15 prior to entry.

Standardized examinations: Graduate Record Examination (GRE), general test, is required. Test scores older than 5 years will not be accepted. The mean combined score on the Graduate Record Examination for the class of 2003 was at the 62nd percentile.

Additional requirements and considerations
   Animal/veterinary work experience
   Recommendations (3 required, one by a veterinarian)
   Extracurricular and/or community service activities

Summary of Admission Procedure

Timetable
   Application deadline: October 1
   Date interviews are held: late February–early March
   Date acceptances mailed: March–April
   School begins: late August

Deposit (to hold place in class): none required

119

Deferments: are considered for financial reasons and completion of graduate degrees.

Evaluation criteria

Applicants will be selected based upon ability to successfully complete the program and demonstration of the qualities of a good veterinarian. Academic criteria include undergraduate, science, and 45-hour GPAs, GRE test scores, and rigor of academic program (and quality of graduate program, if applicable). Nonacademic factors include maturity, integrity, compassion, communication skills, and a desire to contribute to society. An interview will be required for residents of Washington, Idaho, and states outside the WICHE region. WICHE applicants are ranked for WICHE funding using the same criteria above minus the interview.

1999–2000 admissions summary *

	Number of Applicants	Number of New Entrants
Washington	164	39
Idaho	41	11
Contract[†]	215	11
Nonresident	673	9
Total:	1,093	70

* Note: see also section under Oregon State University; Oregon residents apply to Oregon State University. Oregon residents should not apply to WSU through VMCAS.

Expenses for the 1999–2000 Academic Year

Tuition and fees

Resident	$8,988.00
Nonresident	
Contract[†]	$8,988.00
Other nonresidents	$22,162.00

† For further information, see the listing of contracting states and provinces.

Dual-Degree Programs

Combined DVM-graduate degree programs are available.

University of Wisconsin

Office of Academic Affairs
School of Veterinary Medicine
2015 Linden Drive West
University of Wisconsin-Madison
Madison WI 53706-1102
Telephone: (608) 263-2525
www.vetmed.wisc.edu.oaa/oaa.html

The University of Wisconsin is located in Madison, the state capital, which has a population of about 190,000. Consistently ranked among the nation's "most livable" cities, its hilly terrain, scattered parks, and woodlands saturate the urban setting with a friendly neighborhood atmosphere. Centered on a narrow isthmus among 4 scenic lakes, the city is a recreational paradise. The university sprawls over 900 acres along Lake Mendota and its student population is nearly 45,000. It has rated among the top 10 universities academically since 1910 and is third in the country in volume of research activity.

The School of Veterinary Medicine facility has a modern veterinary teaching hospital, modern equipment, and high-quality lab space for teaching and research. The curriculum provides a broad education in veterinary medicine with learning experiences in food animal medicine and other specialty areas. The school pioneered a unique senior rotation in ambulatory service for fourth-year students where they experience the life and work of a veterinarian specializing in large-animal medicine by working in one of 20 practices near Madison. The school has an outstanding research program with faculty in the forefront. Many faculty members have joint appointments with the College of Agriculture, the Medical School, the Regional Primate Center, the McArdle Cancer Research Institute, the National Wildlife Health Laboratory, and the North Central Dairy Forage Center. These outside links provide research and job opportunities for students.

Application Information

Applications available: May

Application deadline: October 1

Application fee: see VMCAS

Institutional application requirements: $45.00 application fee

Residency implications: between 60 and 70 Wisconsin residents will be accepted.

Wisconsin has no contractual agreements, but may accept 10-20 nonresidents. Applicants who can claim legal residency or domicile in more than one state should contact the school. Wisconsin has a cooperative agreement with the Pontifical Catholic University of Puerto Rico and the University of Puerto Rico-Mayaguez (UPR-Mayaguez) annually to offer admission to up to 2 students from the Pontifical Catholic University of Puerto Rico and UPR-Mayaguez. Students from Puerto Rico considering applying to the BS/DVM Binary Program should contact the College of Sciences, Pontifical Catholic University of Puerto Rico, Estacion 6, Ponce, Puerto Rico 00732 and/or the College of Agricultural Sciences, University of Puerto Rico-Mayaguez, P.O. Box 5000, Mayaguez, PR 00681-5000.

Veterinary Medical College Application Service (VMCAS): required for all applicants.

Prerequisites for Admission

Applicants must complete a minimum of 60 semester credits of college coursework. The 60 credits include the required 40-43 credits of coursework listed below, plus a minimum of 17 credits of elective coursework left to the student's discretion. The 17 elective credits allow the student to meet personal and academic goals and objectives while preparing for admission to veterinary school.

Course requirements and semester hours

Biochemistry (organic chemistry must be prerequisite)	3
General biology or zoology, introductory animal biology course (with laboratory)	5
General and qualitative chemistry, 2-semester lecture series (with laboratory)	8
Organic chemistry, 1-semester lecture satisfying biochemistry prerequisite	3
English composition or journalism	6

Must include completion of either of the following:
1. satisfactory score on a college English placement exam, or
2. an introductory English composition course, plus completion of one of the following:
   a. an English composition or journalism course graded on the basis of writing skills, or
   b. written evidence from instructor that writing skills were included in the grading of a specific college-level course

Genetics or animal breeding, must include principles of heredity and preferably molecular mechanisms	3
General physics, 2-semester lecture series	6
Statistics, introductory course	3
Social sciences/humanities, any elective courses in social science or the humanities	6

Required undergraduate GPA: the mean cumulative GPA of the class of 2003 is approximately 3.45 for residents and 3.70 for nonresidents.

AP credit policy: must appear on official college transcripts and be equivalent to the appropriate college-level coursework.

Course completion deadline: all coursework must be completed no later than the spring 2001 term prior to admission to the fall 2001 term.

Standardized examinations: Graduate Record Examination (GRE), general test, is required. The GRE may be taken no later than October 1 in the year of application. The mean score of the class of 2003 for the verbal, quantitative, and analytical portions combined is approximately 1872 for residents and 1942 for nonresidents.

Additional requirements and considerations
    Animal contact and work experience
    Veterinary medical experience
    Other preparatory experience
    College degrees earned
    Extracurricular activities
    Recommendations/evaluations (3 required)
    Scholarships/awards

Summary of Admission Procedure

Timetable
    Application deadline: October 1
    Interviews: none
    Early admission notification: late February (Wisconsin residents)
    Date acceptances mailed: mid-March
    School begins: early September

Deposit (to hold place in class): none required.

Deferments: are considered on an individual basis by the Admissions Committee and may be granted for extenuating circumstances.

Evaluation criteria

There is a 2-part admission procedure. For the fall 1999 admission year, the class was selected based upon the following comparative evaluation:

1. *Evaluation of academic record* (weighted approximately 60 percent)

Undergraduate cumulative GPA

Required course GPA

Most recent 30-45 semester credit GPA

Test scores

2. *Evaluation of personal experience and characteristics*

(weighted approximately 40 percent)

Animal and veterinary work experience

Other preparatory experience (includes extracurricular activities)

Personal history/academic performance (summary category to include review of academic history, academic achievements, diversity of background, etc.)

Reference letters

1999-2000 admissions summary

		Number of Applicants	Number of New Entrants
Resident		179	70
Nonresident		1,151	10
	Total:	1,330	80

Expenses for the 1999-2000 Academic Year

Tuition and fees (estimated)

Resident	$11,362.00
Nonresident	$16,666.00

Dual-Degree Programs

Combined DVM-graduate degree programs are available.

Veterinary Medical Schools in Canada

University of Guelph

Admissions, Office of Registrarial Services
University Centre, Level 3
University of Guelph
Guelph Ontario N1G 2W1
Canada
Telephone: (519) 824-4120, ext. 6062
www.ovc-uoguelph.ca

Founded in 1862, the Ontario Veterinary College is located in Guelph about 60 miles north of Buffalo. Guelph has a similar climate to Detroit and Chicago. Surrounded by gently rolling farmland, this city of 90,000 is typical of the northeast.

The university has an enrollment of 12,220 undergraduate students, of whom 400 are veterinary students. There are also approximately 150 graduate students, 100 faculty, and 200 staff members at the veterinary college, which offers degree programs leading to a DVM, MS, PhD, Doctor of Veterinary Science (DVSc) and a Graduate Diploma. The college has 4 departments— Population Medicine, Clinical Studies, Biomedical Sciences, and Pathobiology —and a full-service teaching hospital. Funding for research comes from 2 sources: the Ontario Ministry of Agriculture, Food and Rural Affairs research contract of 4.6 million $C and external research grants and contracts of 3.9 million $C. There are also large, modern research stations for separately housing sheep, swine, and dairy and beef cattle.

Application Information

Applications available: September

Application deadline: October 1—VMCAS; December 1 all others

Application fee: 90.00 $C

Residency implications: Canadian citizens or individuals who have permanent resident status of at least one year's duration who are residents of Ontario will be considered. International applicants will be considered provided the applicant does not hold Canadian citizenship or permanent resident status in Canada. There is a maximum of 5 international positions available per year.

Veterinary Medical College Application Service (VMCAS): optional for international (non-Canadian) residents.

Prerequisites for Admission

Course requirements and semester hours: Students must first complete a minimum of two full-time years (four full-time semesters) of university including specific university courses. Students initially apply for admission to a science degree program. For the purpose of DVM admission, a full-time semester will include at least 5 one-semester courses. Once the prerequisite courses are completed successfully, students apply for admission to the DVM Program.

Effective September 2000 Admission: The subject matter requirements listed below must have been completed before admission to the DVM program will be considered.

Course requirements and semesters

Biological sciences (emphasis on animal biology; one semester must be cell biology)	3
Genetics	1
Biochemistry	1
Statistics (with a university-level calculus prerequisite)	1
Humanities or social sciences*	2

* Students entering the DVM program should be able to operate across discipline boundaries recognizing the relevance of the humanities and social sciences to their career choice. In selecting these courses from among those acceptable, the prospective veterinary student should consider topics such as ethics, logic, critical thinking, determinants of human behavior, and human social interaction.

Required courses proposed to be completed at an institution other than the University of Guelph should be approved as acceptable prior to registration. Applicants are required to request approval for courses in writing. Course descriptions *must* be included with the request. Courses will *not* be acceptable if they are repeats of previously passed courses, or if they are taken at the same or a lower level in a subject area than previously passed courses in the same subject area. It is expected that the required undergraduate preparation for the DVM program will be completed in a full-time coherent academic program.

Required undergraduate GPA: students with a minimum A (80% — GPA 3.60) based on the average of the required courses and the last 2 semesters in full-time attendance at university may be further considered.

Course completion deadline: required courses must be completed by June 15 of the year of application in order to be further considered.

Standardized examinations: Medical College Admission Test (MCAT) is required. Test scores must be received no later than December 1 of the year of application.

Additional requirements and considerations
　　Reasons for choosing a career in veterinary medicine
　　Quality of preparatory academic program
　　Experience and knowledge in matters relating to animals and to the veterinary medical profession
　　Experience and achievement in extracurricular affairs and/or community service activities
　　Communication skills
　　Referees' reports

Summary of Admission Procedure

Timetable
　　Application deadline: October 1 for VMCAS applications; December 1 for all others
　　Date interviews are held: February–June
　　Date acceptances mailed: March–July
　　School begins: September

Deposit (to hold place in class): $500.00

1999–2000 admissions summary

	Number of Applicants	Number of New Entrants
Residents	550	100
International Residents	100	5
Total:	650	105

Expenses for the 1999-2000 Academic Year

Tuition and fees
　　Resident　　　　　　　　　　$4,500.00 $C
　　Visa student　　　　　　　　$35,000.00 $C

Université de Montréal

Service des Admissions
Université de Montréal
C.P. 6205
Succursale Centre-Ville
Montréal Québec H3C 3T5
Canada
Téléphone: (514) 343-7076
E-mail: saefmv@medvet.umontreal.ca
www.medvet.umontreal.ca

Renseignements pour les applications/Application Information

Formulaires disponibles dès: décembre
Applications available: December

Date limite de remise: 1er mars
Application deadline: March 1

Frais d'application: 30.00 $C
Application fee: 30.00 $C

Statut de résident: Il faut être citoyen Canadien ou résident permanent pour être admissible.
Residency implications: Canadian citizenship or permanent residency in Canada is required.

Prérequis/Prerequisites for Admission

DEC (Diplôme d'Etudes Collégiales) en sciences de la nature
DEC (Junior College Diploma: obtained in Quebec) majoring in nature science. (The DEC represents 2 years of post-high school studies.)

Cours/Course requirements

Physique/Physics	101, 201, 301–78
Chimie/Chemistry	101, 201, 202
Biologie/Biology	301, 401
Mathématiques (avec calcul intégral)/ Mathematics (including calculus)	103, 203

Pour être admis au programme de DMV, il faut: a) avoir satisfait les conditions ci-dessus, ou b) faire preuve d'études équivalentes.

To be considered for admission, one must: a) have completed the above requirements, or b) have completed equivalent studies.

Note: All lectures are given in French. Examinations must be written in French.

Le programme de DMV est maintenant réparti sur cinq ans.

The DMV is now a 5-year program.

La Maîtrise de la langue française est une condition de diplômation. Par conséquent, tout nouvel étudiant doit réussir le test de français du Ministère de l'Education ou, s'il échoue au test, réussir les cours de français prescrits par l'Université.

Language requirements: All students entering undergraduate degree programs must show that they have mastery of the French language in order to qualify for the degree. This graduation requirement may be met either by passing the Quebec Department of Education French test or by passing designated remedial French courses.

Test de Français: Le succès à ce test n'est pas obligatoire pour l'admission mais l'étudiant doit le réussir pour obtenir son diplôme.

French test: Success in passing this language test is not a prerequisite for admission in first year of the veterinary program, but each student must pass the test successfully to earn a diploma.

Performance Score: This score is obtained by comparing the student's grade in each course with the class average.

Dossier academique avant admission: Le candidat doit, ou bien avoir terminé, ou s'être inscrit à tous les cours prérequis au moment de l'application.

Course completion deadline: The applicant must be registered for or have completed all prerequisites at the time of application.

Critères de sélection (priorité d'importance)/Additional considerations (in order of importance)
1. Dossier académique
2. Entrevue: l'entrevue a été structurée pour évaluer la motivation, la préparation et le raisonnement des candidats.
1. Academic record
2. Interview: the interview is designed to verify the applicant's motivation, preparation, judgment, etc. The above list reflects priorities (applicants are judged first on academic merit, then test/exam results, etc.).

Cédule du processus/Summary of Admission Procedure

Horaire
    Date limite de remise des formules: le 1er mars
    Entrevues: mi-mai
    Notification d'acceptation: fin mai, début juin
    Début de l'année scolaire: fin août

Timetable
    Application deadline: March 1
    Interviews: mid-May
    Notification of acceptance: end of May, early June
    Fall semester begins: end of August

Dépôt nécessaire pour garder une place dans la classe: aucun.
Deposit (to hold place in class): none required.

L'acceptation ne peut, en aucun cas, être reportée à une année subséquente.
Deferments: not considered.

Critères d'évaluation/Evaluation criteria	%
Résultats scolaires/Performance score	60
Entrevue/Interview	40

Budget estimé/Estimated Expenses for the 1999-2000 Academic Year

Frais de scolarité:	55.61 $C	par credit (approx. 50 credits par année)
Tuition and fees:	55.61 $C	per credit (approx. 50 per year)

University of Prince Edward Island

Registrar's Office
Atlantic Veterinary College
University of Prince Edward Island
550 University Avenue
Charlottetown PEI C1A 4P3
Canada
Telephone: (902) 566-0608
E-mail: registrar@upei.ca
www.upei.ca/~regoff/

The Atlantic Veterinary College (AVC), one of the newest colleges of veterinary medicine in North America, was completed in 1987 and is fully accredited by the American Veterinary Medical Association, the Canadian Veterinary Medical Association, and the Royal College of Veterinary Surgeons (UK).

Centrally located on Canada's eastern seaboard (650 miles northeast of Boston), the Atlantic Veterinary College makes its home in a beautiful island setting in Charlottetown, Prince Edward Island. With a population of 135,000, which jumps to over a million during the summer tourist season, the community enjoys a small-town lifestyle that boasts the amenities of larger cities, including dining and theatre. Residents also enjoy outdoor activities, such as golfing, cycling, sailing, and cross-country skiing.

The college is a completely integrated teaching, research, and service facility. The four-story complex contains the veterinary teaching hospital, diagnostic services, fish health unit, farm services, postmortem services, animal barns, laboratories, classrooms, computer and audio-visual facilities, offices, cafeteria, and study areas. The Atlantic Veterinary College also operates a nearby farm facility, a swine research facility, and a fish hatchery.

Prince Edward Island is a scenic province with a wide variety of dairy, beef, hog, sheep, horse, and fish farms. The combination and variety of animal and fish farms have allowed AVC to develop a special expertise in fish health, aquaculture, and population medicine.

Application Information

Applications available: May — VMCAS; September — institutional

Application deadline: October 1 for VMCAS applicants; December 1 for all others

Institutional application requirements: 35.00 $C; $50.00 (U.S.) for VMCAS applicants

Residency implications: Atlantic Veterinary College currently has contracts with New Brunswick (13), Newfoundland (2), Nova Scotia (16), and the home province P.E.I. (10). International students are admitted on a noncontract basis (19).

Veterinary Medical College Application Service (VMCAS): required for U.S. citizens or residents; optional for non-U.S. international (non-Canadian) residents.

Prerequisites for Admission

The preveterinary program leading to admission at the Atlantic Veterinary College will normally take 2 years to complete.

Course requirements
The equivalent of 20 one-semester courses are required, including:
  Mathematics, 2 courses, including statistics
  Biology, 4 courses, including genetics and microbiology
  Chemistry, 3 courses, including organic chemistry
  Physics, 1 course
  English, 2 courses, one of which must be a course in English composition
  Humanities and social sciences, 3 courses
  Electives, 5 courses from any discipline
  (Science courses will normally have a laboratory component.)

Required undergraduate GPA: no minimum stated; mean cumulative GPA of most recent entering class is 3.14 on a 4.00 scale.

AP credit policy: not accepted.

Course completion deadline: June 1 of the year of application.

Standardized examinations: Graduate Record Examination (GRE) (for non-Canadian applicants only). If a student's native language or language of prior education is not English, then the student will be required to pass one of the following: TOEFL, MELAB, IELB, or CanTest.

Additional requirements and considerations
  Veterinary-related experience: at least two 40-hour experiences with veterinarians in practice, government, industry, or in a research environment at an academic institution are required. One of these experiences must involve clinical practice in the field. If an applicant selects 2 clinical experiences, he or she cannot be in the same field or under the supervision of the same veterinarian.
  Veterinary evaluations

Interview
Essay
Additional academic achievement
Recommendations/evaluations not required

Summary of Admission Procedure

Timetable

Application deadline: October 1 for VMCAS applications; December 1 for all others

Date interviews are held: April

Date acceptances mailed: mid-July

School begins: late August–early September; registration, early September

Deposit (to hold place in class): none required.

Deferments: are considered for extenuating circumstances.

Evaluation criteria

Academic credentials and animal work experience are objectively evaluated by the Registrar's Office. Other criteria and activities are subjectively evaluated by the admissions committee through an interview process.

	% weight
Grades	50
Additional academic achievement	5
Veterinary experience, interview	35
Essay	10

1999–2000 admissions summary

	Number of Applicants	Number of New Entrants
In-province	32	10
Contract*	120	30
International	438	20
Total:	590	60

Expenses for the 2000-2001 Academic Year

Tuition and fees

Resident	6,770.00 $C
Contract student*	6,770.00 $C
International student	39,200.00 $C

* For further information, see the listing of contracting states and provinces.

University of Saskatchewan

Admissions Office
Western College of Veterinary Medicine
52 Campus Drive
University of Saskatchewan
Saskatoon Saskatchewan S7N 5B4
Canada
Telephone: (306) 966-7454
www.usask.ca/wcvm

The Western College of Veterinary Medicine is located in the city of Saskatoon, which has a population of about 180,000 and is the major urban center in central Saskatchewan. The city is also the major commercial center for central and northern Saskatchewan and is served by 2 national airlines with direct connections to all major centers in Canada. Summers are short and cool; winters are long and cold.

The Western College of Veterinary Medicine is one of the few veterinary colleges where all health sciences and agriculture are offered on the same campus. The college is devoted to undergraduate education and has a reputation in Canada and in the northwestern United States for educating veterinarians who are well-rounded in general veterinary medicine and have good practical backgrounds. It has one of the best field-service caseloads in North America.

Application Information

Applications available: October

Application deadline: January 3

Application fee: 50.00 $C

Residency implications: students are selected for quota positions from Alberta, British Columbia, Manitoba, the Northwest Territories, Saskatchewan, and the Yukon Territory. Occasional positions are available to other Canadian residents. Special consideration is given to self-identified individuals of aboriginal origin. Residents of foreign countries where veterinary schools exist are not considered.

Veterinary Medical College Application Service (VMCAS): no participation.

Prerequisites for Admission

Course requirements and semester hours

English	6
Physics	6
Biology	6
Genetics	3
Introductory chemistry	6
Organic chemistry	3
Mathematics or statistics	6
Biochemistry	6
Microbiology	3
Electives	15

Required undergraduate GPA: a minimum cumulative average of 70% is required.

Course completion deadline: prerequisite courses must be completed by the time of entry into the program.

Standardized examinations: none required.

Additional requirements and considerations
Animal/veterinary work experience, motivation, and knowledge
Maturity
Leadership
Communication skills

Summary of Admission Procedure

Timetable
Application deadline: January 3
Date interviews are held: May–June
Date acceptances mailed: on or before July 1
School begins: late August

Deposit (to hold place in class): none required.

Deferments: not considered.

Evaluation criteria

The 3-part admission procedure consists of an assessment of academic ability, a personal interview, and an overall assessment of the application file.

	% weight
Grades	60
Interview*	30
Judgment	10

* Interview selection is based entirely on academic performance.

1999–2000 admissions summary

	Number of Applicants	*Number of New Entrants*
Resident	50	20
Contract†	261	50
Nonresident	16	0
Total:	317	70

Expenses for the 1999–2000 Academic Year

Tuition and fees

Resident	5,107.00 $C
Nonresident	
Contract student†	5,107.00 $C
Other nonresident-Canadian	5,107.00 $C

† For further information, see the listing of contracting states and provinces.

Policies on Advanced Standing

Transfers are permitted to most colleges of veterinary medicine in the United States under specified conditions. Typical requirements include a vacancy in the class, completion of all prerequisite requirements, and compatible curricula. Following is a listing of schools and some of the conditions under which they will consider a transfer from another veterinary college with advanced standing. More detailed information may be obtained by writing to the individual schools in which you have an interest.

UNITED STATES

University of California

1. An opening must exist in the second- or third-year class.
2. The applicant must have completed equivalent coursework to that of students in the class to which that person seeks admission.
3. The applicant must meet the minimum academic requirements for admission as stated in the Guide for Prospective Students.
4. Priority is given to California residents. It is usually not possible to determine if a position will be available until after July 1 in any given year.

Colorado State University

Advanced standing will be considered on an individual basis subject to the following provisions:

1. An open position must be available within the applicable tuition classification category for an additional student.
2. The applicant must meet all prerequisites for admission to the program as a first-year student and possess qualifications that are competitive with currently enrolled students.
3. The applicant must have completed at least one full academic year at the institution in which currently enrolled and have achieved a cumulative GPA of 3.00 or better (of 4.00) and be in good academic standing. Transfer credit will not be allowed for any course receiving a grade of less than 2.00 (of 4.00).
4. If the applicant is acceptable to the Admissions Committee and a position is available, placement will be offered in the year and term of the curriculum deemed appropriate after analysis of equivalency of the required courses.
5. Applicant must be enrolled in an AVMA accredited college.

Students attending non-AVMA accredited institutions must apply for admission to the first-year class through the regular admissions process.

University of Florida

1. An opening must exist in the second- or third-year class.
2. Students with advanced standing are rarely considered for admission to second- or third-year classes on the basis of exceptional personal circumstances.
3. Student must be enrolled in an AVMA accredited college.
4. Student must meet all prerequisites for admission as a first-year student (including GRE scores).
5. The curricula of the two schools must be sufficiently alike to allow a student to enter without deficiencies in academic background.
6. Applicant must *not* have been denied admission to the University of Florida College of Veterinary Medicine as a first-year student.
7. Applicants must have a letter approving transfer from their dean or associate dean.

University of Georgia

1. Must be a resident of the United States, with priority given to Georgia residents, followed by contract state residents, then all other citizens.
2. Applicants will be considered for entry up to the third year.
3. Applications must include a letter of support written and submitted by the dean of the school in which the applicant is currently enrolled.
4. All selection criteria for regular applicants apply to transfer applicants.
5. No individual is eligible for transfer who has been dismissed or is on probation at any other school or college for deficiency in scholarship or because of misconduct.

University of Illinois

1. Requests for transfer are considered on a case-by-case basis to maintain class size.
2. All prerequisite science courses must be completed prior to the request for transfer.
3. Minimum grade requirements include:
   cumulative and science GPAs of 2.75 on a 4.00 scale;
   semester GPA of 2.25 on a 4.00 scale for each semester of veterinary medical coursework completed (all undergraduate and current veterinary school);
   courses must be completed with a grade of C– or better (2.00 = C).

4. Student must complete the same preveterinary coursework as required for all students accepted to the program.
5. Student must be in good academic standing.
6. To request transfer consideration, student must submit a letter explaining the reasons for transfer, official transcripts from all universities/colleges attended, description of all veterinary coursework completed to date, and a letter from the dean of the current school certifying the applicant's academic standing.

Iowa State University

1. The applicant must have had essentially the same preveterinary coursework as required of Iowa State students and must have met the minimum qualifications of those admitted to the College of Veterinary Medicine.
2. The applicant must have completed the equivalent of all courses required of Iowa State University veterinary students beginning the academic term the applicant seeks to enter. Only credits earned at an AVMA accredited college of veterinary medicine will be considered for credit.
3. The applicant must have been in good standing throughout his or her entire period of enrollment in the school(s) of veterinary medicine in which the student is, or has been, enrolled. A letter to that effect from the dean(s) of the school(s) is required.
4. Space must be available.

Kansas State University

Acceptance of students for advanced standing is on recommendation of the Admissions Committee on a space-available basis.

Louisiana State University

Applicants must have successfully completed all previous professional courses in an AVMA accredited college or school of veterinary medicine. The request for transfer and supporting documents are reviewed by the Committee on Admissions. After review the committee forwards a recommendation to the dean for approval or denial of the transfer request.

Michigan State University

1. Admission consideration is offered only to those current matriculants in professional veterinary curricula who believe that there are extenuating circumstances that would precipitate significant undue hardship if they continue at their current institution.

2. Applicants must also demonstrate quality academic performance throughout their professional school enrollment.
3. The curricula of the two schools must be sufficiently alike to allow a student to enter the second-year class without deficiencies in academic background.
4. All selection criteria for regular applicants apply to transfer applicants.
5. Priority is given to Michigan residents.
6. AVMA accreditation of current school is considered.

University of Minnesota

1. Transfers are not allowed to any specific requested year or semester. The committee will place each applicant in the year or semester of the curriculum deemed appropriate after analysis of equivalency of the required courses involved.
2. No academic work or standing will be accepted from DVM curricula other than those deemed accredited ("AVMA accredited") or approved ("AVMA approved") by the American Veterinary Medical Association.
3. All applicants must be U.S. citizens, be holders of permanent resident alien visas, or have achieved landed immigrant status.
4. All applicants are required to have finished at least one full academic year at the institution from which transfer is requested and must be in good academic standing at the time of discontinuance according to written verification from the institution.
5. All applicants must document that not more than two calendar years have elapsed between discontinuance and application to our DVM program.
6. All applicants must have achieved a cumulative GPA of 3.00 (of 4.00) for the required courses at the initial institution.
7. All applicants must present suitable transcripts and course summary descriptions of all courses taken. These must be carried to the appropriate course coordinator in our curriculum, and each coordinator must certify in writing that the transfer courses satisfy our curricular specifications according to comparative criteria determined by each coordinator in discussion with the petitioner. The applicant is responsible for preparing a standard University of Minnesota Petition Form, obtaining the course instructor's dated signature, and returning it to the Office for Student Affairs and Admission. If equivalency is not certified, the course must be taken in our curriculum prior to the transfer to a specific veterinary class year.

Mississippi State University

A limited number of transfer students are accepted in order to maintain a stable class size. Transfer positions are filled on a competitive basis.

1. Applicants must attend an interview at the College of Veterinary Medicine to be eligible for admission.
2. Applicants must submit complete transcripts of all DVM coursework.
3. Transfers are limited to the first two years of the curriculum. No student can transfer into the curriculum beyond the start of the third year of the professional program.
4. Candidates must demonstrate quality academic performance and professional behavior to be considered for transfer. Transfer applicants who have failed one or more courses at another college of veterinary medicine will not be considered for admission. Transfer applicants who have been dismissed for academic or other reasons from any other college of veterinary medicine will not be considered for admission.
5. To initiate transfer, candidates must submit a formal letter of intent, stating reasons for transfer, and an official transcript from their professional program.

University of Missouri

1. Must be a vacancy in the class.
2. Will consider students who are U.S. citizens or holders of permanent alien visas and who have finished at least two years in a college of veterinary medicine that is AVMA accredited.
3. Students must be in good academic standing, and a letter of reference from the dean's office of the present college is required.

North Carolina State University

1. Must be a vacancy in the class.
2. Consideration by the Admission Committee on an individual basis.
3. Curricula must be compatible.
4. Support letter required from the dean's office.
5. Letter of recommendation from a faculty member at the original college.
6. Only accept transfers from AVMA accredited colleges.
7. At least 50% of DVM credit hours should be completed at North Carolina State in order to earn a North Carolina State degree.

Ohio State University

1. An opening must exist.
2. Student must be enrolled in an AVMA accredited college.

3. The curricula of the two schools must be sufficiently alike to allow the student to enter a class without deficiencies in his or her academic background.
4. Student must be in good academic standing in present college and have a supporting letter from the Dean of Student and Academic Affairs to this effect.
5. Each request for transfer is considered on an individual basis, taking into account personal hardship, family situations, etc.
6. Must meet same prerequisite requirements as first-year applicants.

Oklahoma State University

1. A student will normally enter at the beginning of the fall semester, second year, regardless of his/her standing at the school from which he/she is transferring.
2. A student may be accepted only if a vacancy exists in the second-year class, fall semester.
3. Preference will be given to students from schools/colleges with AVMA accreditation.
4. Application deadline is April 15, with all requirements having been met prior to entry date.
5. Applications accepted only from students from institutions that are accredited by an authentic accrediting agency.

Oregon State University

Admission of students with advanced standing is considered only in very specific and unique circumstances, and each case is considered on an individual basis.

University of Pennsylvania

1. An opening must exist.
2. Admission with Advanced Standing (AAS) is considered only from institutions that are accredited by the AVMA.
3. Student must initiate the process at his/her own institution. The Dean of Student Affairs at the college from which the student wants to transfer must understand the student's need for AAS and endorse it. The usual reasons endorsed are either medical or the desire to move nearer one's spouse.
4. If the Dean of Student Affairs approves, student must send detailed description of all coursework taken to date and simultaneously submit an application to the University of Pennsylvania's Admissions Committee. If the

Admissions Committee accepts the credentials, it will compare coursework with that of the University of Pennsylvania and determine where in the curriculum the student might be placed.

5. If all criteria are met and space is available, AAS may be granted.
6. University of Pennsylvania cannot award a degree to a student who has completed less than 50% of graduation credits at Penn.

Purdue University

1. Must be a vacancy in the class.
2. Curricula must be compatible.
3. Must be in good academic standing at present college.
4. Must have an acceptable undergraduate record as determined by the Admissions Committee.
5. Admission limited to the first or second year of the program.

University of Tennessee

Admission of students with advanced standing may be considered for unique circumstances on a case-by-case basis. Space must be available in the class and the professional curricula must reasonably match between the schools. The Admissions Committee will review applicants' credentials and interview those determined to best meet their criteria. Admission is usually limited to the second semester of the first year of the professional curriculum. Students must be in good standing at their present college.

Texas A & M University

Students requesting advanced standing must meet the following requirements:

1. Must have completed all previous professional veterinary courses in an AVMA accredited college of veterinary medicine.
2. Must have successfully completed the academic term preceding the semester into which student requests admission.
3. Must comply with all requirements for transfer into the university as described in the current catalog.
4. May request transfer only into the second through seventh semesters of the professional curriculum.
5. At the time of matriculation the student must certify by letter that he/she has not been convicted of crimes in the period from first enrollment in the college of veterinary medicine from which the student desires transfer until date of matriculation at Texas A&M University.
6. To request transfer consideration, the student must:

submit a letter explaining the reason(s) for requesting transfer, desired date of transfer, and class and semester of curriculum into which transfer is requested; and provide a letter of character and academic reference (including class ranking) from the dean of the college from which student desires the transfer; two letters of reference from former instructors who are members of the faculty of the college from which student desires the transfer; and official copies of all academic transcripts.

Tufts University

Applicants from other veterinary schools are considered. Students with advanced standing are admitted if and when space becomes available in the second- or third-year class. The application deadline is June 1 for the following September.

Virginia Polytechnic Institute and State University

1. Applicants may be a Virginia or Maryland resident or a nonresident enrolled in another veterinary school.
2. Advanced standing is allowed only if a vacancy exists. Class size cannot exceed 90 students. Must start at the beginning of second or third year.
3. Must have a 3.00 GPA in veterinary school attended.
4. Must submit transcripts from all colleges attended and meet minimum GPA requirements for all college work.
5. Must have completed the same preprofessional courses required for first-year admission with a grade of C- or higher.
6. Must have prevet credentials that would have resulted in an offer of admission or placement on the alternate list for a position in the class/year being requested.
7. Letters from current dean and two faculty members are required.
8. Petition for advanced standing, with reasons for same, must be received by May 1 of the year in which transfer occurs.

Washington State University

Admission of students with advanced standing is effected only in very specific and unique circumstances, and each case is considered on an individual basis.

University of Wisconsin

Requests will be evaluated using the same selection criteria established for applicants to the first-year class and will be considered under the following circumstances:

1. Applicant will be considered for admission only if there is space available in the class into which he/she wishes to enter.
2. The applicant must have attended an AVMA accredited college of veterinary medicine.
3. Applicant must have passed all professional courses and attained the minimum cumulative GPA required for promotion of students.
4. Wisconsin residents will be given first consideration for admission if the above criteria have been met.

CANADA

University of Guelph
Admission with advanced standing from other veterinary schools will be considered provided a vacancy exists and the applicant can fulfill the residence requirements and has a satisfactory academic record. The occurrence of vacancies is extremely rare.

University of Prince Edward Island
Applicants who have completed all or portions of a veterinary medical program may apply for advanced standing to the second year of the DVM program. Applicants for advanced standing must present evidence of educational accomplishments and may be required to satisfactorily pass examinations in all of the courses for which they desire credit. Students admitted with advanced standing must begin the college year in September.

The candidate must file a formal application and may be interviewed by the Admissions Committee and possibly other faculty. Places for admission to the college with advanced standing are limited and depend on vacancies.

It is imperative that the Admissions Committee have detailed and translated summaries of veterinary medical academic programs and accomplishments for those seeking advanced placement from schools in foreign countries. Advanced-standing applications should be on file and completed as early as possible and no later than January 1.

University of Saskatchewan
1. Must have a vacancy.
2. Curricula must be compatible.
3. Residency requirements apply.
4. There is no admission beyond the second year.
5. GRE is required.
6. TOEFL is required if first language is not English.

Application and Enrollment Data

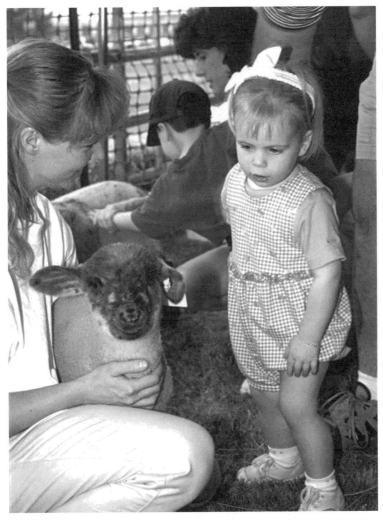

Visitors of all ages enjoy the annual Open House at Auburn University's College of Veterinary Medicine. Photo courtesy Auburn University College of Veterinary Medicine.

Table 1
Applications and Applicants to Colleges of Veterinary Medicine, 1977-99

Year	Number of Colleges	First Year Positions	Number of Applications	Applications per Position	Applicants
1977	22	1,973	10,704	5.43	—
1978	22	2,086	9,467	4.54	—
1979	24	2,296	10,120	4.41	—
1980	25	2,213	9,525	4.30	7,286
1981	26	2,220	8,367	3.65	6,373
1982	26	2,231	8,262	3.70	6,182
1983*	27	2,306	8,074	3.50	5,805
1984	27	2,300	8,291	3.60	5,503
1985	27	2,282	7,953	3.49	4,961
1986	27	2,277	7,719	3.39	4,751
1987	27	2,199	7,729	3.51	4,432
1988	27	2,195	7,422	3.38	4,200
1989	27	2,189	7,098	3.24	3,922
1990	27	2,191	7,218	3.29	3,955
1991	27	2,172	7,848	3.61	4,296
1992	27	2,317	8,737	3.77	4,709
1993	27	2,309	9,939	4.30	4,957
1994	27	2,314	10,961	4.74	5,428
1995	27	2,290	12,499	5.46	6,634
1996†	27	2,322	22,578	9.72	6,424
1997	27	2,302	23,595	10.25	6,630
1998	27	2,330	27,312	11.72	6,783
1999	27	2,301	24,448	10.62	6,695

* Data for 1983 may be inconsistent due to incomplete reporting from two colleges.
† Year 1 of VMCAS operations

Table 2
Acceptance of First-Time and Repeat Applicants, 1995-99

Applicants	1995			1996		
	Total Number	Number Accepted	Percent Accepted	Total Number	Number Accepted	Percent Accepted
First-time	4,879	1,714	35.1	4,740	1,740	36.7
Repeat	1,755	566	32.3	1,684	553	32.8
Total	6,634	2,280	34.4	6,424	2,293	35.7

Applicants per Position	Percentage Accepted*	Applications per Applicant	Repeat Applicants	New Applicants
–	–	–	–	–
–	–	–	–	–
–	–	–	–	–
3.29	30.40	1.31	–	–
2.87	34.80	1.31	–	–
2.77	36.10	1.34	–	–
2.52	39.80	1.39	2,121	3,684
2.39	41.80	1.51	1,842	3,661
2.17	46.00	1.60	1,660	3,301
2.09	47.93	1.62	1,394	3,357
2.02	49.62	1.74	1,252	3,180
1.91	52.26	1.77	1,095	3,105
1.79	55.81	1.81	984	2,938
1.81	55.40	1.83	862	3,093
1.98	50.56	1.83	861	3,435
2.03	49.20	1.86	960	3,749
2.15	46.58	2.01	1,117	3,840
2.35	42.63	2.02	1,380	4,048
2.89	34.40	1.88	1,755	4,879
2.77	35.70	3.51	1,684	4,740
2.88	33.29	3.56	1,930	4,700
2.91	32.27	4.03	2,306	4,477
2.91	32.83	3.65	2,366	4,329

1997			1998			1999		
Total Number	Number Accepted	Percent Accepted	Total Number	Number Accepted	Percent Accepted	Total Number	Number Accepted	Percent Accepted
4,700	1,654	35.19	4,477	1,528	34.13	4,329	1,521	35.14
1,930	553	28.65	2,306	661	28.66	2,366	677	28.61
6,630	2,207	33.29	6,783	2,189	32.27	6,695	2,198	32.83

Table 3

Applications per Position in Entering Class in U.S. Colleges of Veterinary Medicine, 1995-99

College	1995 A	P	A/P	1996 A	P	A/P
Auburn Univ	446	92	4.85	917	90	10.19
Univ of California	552	108	5.11	736	109	6.75
Colorado State	764	132	5.79	746	134	5.57
Cornell Univ	622	82	7.59	732	80	9.15
Univ of Florida	487	80	6.09	766	80	9.58
Univ of Georgia	431	87	4.95	763	92	8.29
Univ of Illinois	379	87	4.36	736	87	8.46
Iowa State	690	100	6.90	1,773	102	17.38
Kansas State	341	107	3.19	559	107	5.22
Louisiana State	371	80	4.64	1,075	80	13.44
Michigan State	554	100	5.54	1,375	111	12.39
Univ of Minnesota	489	76	6.43	1,168	76	15.37
Mississippi State	167	49	3.41	340	49	6.94
Univ of Missouri	295	64	4.61	254	64	3.97
North Carolina State	500	78	6.41	1,021	72	14.18
Ohio State	423	133	3.18	478	133	3.59
Oklahoma State	411	71	5.79	682	74	9.22
Oregon State	324	36	9.00	892	36	24.78
Univ of Pennsylvania	744	109	6.83	1,307	105	12.45
Purdue Univ	506	69	7.33	925	65	14.23
Univ of Tennessee	334	63	5.30	566	68	8.32
Texas A&M	431	128	3.37	591	128	4.62
Tufts Univ	685	75	9.13	672	79	8.51
Tuskegee Univ	208	62	3.35	267	61	4.38
VA-MD Regional	249	80	3.11	560	90	6.22
Washington State	502	62	8.10	1,202	70	17.17
Univ of Wisconsin	594	80	7.43	1,475	80	18.44
Total	12,499	2,290	5.46	22,578	2,322	9.72

A = Applications
P = Positions in entering class as reported in this survey
A/P = Applications received per position

1997			1998			1999		
A	*P*	*A/P*	*A*	*P*	*A/P*	*A*	*P*	*A/P*
877	90	9.74	934	90	10.38	819	90	9.10
814	108	7.54	1,134	109	10.40	1,058	108	9.80
758	134	5.66	804	134	6.00	845	133	6.35
1,178	82	14.37	1,517	82	18.50	1,239	81	15.30
745	80	9.31	853	80	10.66	812	80	10.15
681	80	8.51	831	92	9.03	820	81	10.12
481	101	4.76	1,264	101	12.51	1,073	100	10.73
1,665	100	16.65	1,787	102	17.52	1,126	100	11.26
737	100	7.37	1,278	100	12.78	728	100	7.28
1,073	80	13.41	1,284	80	16.05	1,144	80	14.30
1,218	100	12.18	1,324	111	11.93	1,317	101	13.04
1,174	76	15.45	1,155	76	15.20	1,036	76	13.63
336	49	6.86	415	49	8.47	466	49	9.51
232	64	3.63	238	64	3.72	221	64	3.45
1,084	72	15.06	1,162	72	16.14	1,150	72	15.97
1,122	135	8.31	1,048	133	7.88	1,012	133	7.61
638	70	9.11	635	74	8.58	470	74	6.35
964	36	26.78	1,167	36	32.42	986	37	26.65
1,203	110	10.94	1,354	110	12.31	1,378	107	12.88
852	60	14.20	1,000	60	16.67	947	60	15.78
589	68	8.66	606	68	8.91	463	68	6.81
1,010	128	7.89	1,082	128	8.45	955	128	7.46
714	79	9.04	698	79	8.84	759	79	9.61
298	60	4.97	263	60	4.38	216	60	3.60
750	90	8.33	951	90	10.57	992	90	11.02
1,105	70	15.79	1,160	70	16.57	1,090	70	15.57
1,297	80	16.21	1,368	80	17.10	1,326	80	16.58
23,595	2,302	10.25	27,312	2,330	11.72	24,448	2,301	10.62

Table 4

Applicants to U.S. Colleges of Veterinary Medicine by Residence, 1989-99

Residence	1989	1990	1991	1992	1993	1994
Alabama	117	122	116	124	129	135
Alaska	13	11	14	17	15	11
Arizona	30	35	51	50	59	70
Arkansas	26	25	30	30	44	30
California	377	353	409	439	386	434
Colorado	142	143	174	203	230	274
Connecticut	54	47	50	24	46	57
Delaware	7	7	13	9	13	9
Dist. of Col.	—	4	—	1	—	5
Florida	165	144	143	176	188	197
Georgia	109	90	112	136	134	153
Hawaii	17	21	16	16	18	18
Idaho	16	19	27	31	31	38
Illinois	149	184	185	209	210	233
Indiana	75	74	91	117	111	116
Iowa	83	110	135	81	130	95
Kansas	75	53	66	90	88	99
Kentucky	44	53	71	80	97	93
Louisiana	60	66	81	83	93	99
Maine	12	14	16	11	16	24
Maryland	90	87	87	105	107	156
Massachusetts	121	95	102	106	100	153
Michigan	151	165	149	181	140	175
Minnesota	67	79	91	96	112	104
Mississippi	67	61	60	55	37	43
Missouri	77	69	78	96	91	121
Montana	25	20	24	24	18	31
Nebraska	27	33	41	45	48	61
Nevada	25	10	14	13	16	22
New Hampshire	11	12	15	24	22	20
New Jersey	99	103	106	126	94	97

Due to multiple sources of data for each applicant, the total count per state may exceed the total number of applicants.

1995	1996	1997	1998	1999	% Change 1989-99	% Change 1998-99
153	134	152	169	153	30.8	-9.5
11	26	5	13	7	-46.2	-46.2
101	83	70	63	74	146.7	17.5
43	41	30	53	36	38.5	-32.1
545	495	524	553	538	42.7	-2.7
300	297	328	337	350	146.5	3.9
94	61	61	48	50	-7.4	4.2
13	16	13	13	18	157.1	38.5
7	7	4	5	1	—	-80.0
239	258	289	276	265	60.6	-4.0
194	199	207	214	239	119.3	11.7
30	19	27	24	24	41.2	—
46	33	42	43	41	156.3	-4.7
261	238	221	255	263	76.5	3.1
133	125	119	122	126	68.0	3.3
110	154	177	156	128	54.2	-17.9
91	115	121	97	118	57.3	21.6
97	92	122	113	102	131.8	-9.7
114	129	197	201	202	236.7	0.5
54	22	20	15	11	-8.3	-26.7
119	119	130	132	144	60.0	9.1
220	178	182	171	182	50.4	6.4
209	230	249	259	226	49.7	-12.7
177	135	136	145	137	104.5	-5.5
50	57	91	83	79	17.9	-4.8
132	129	143	146	158	105.2	8.2
32	32	34	45	39	56.0	-13.3
60	66	85	70	65	140.7	-7.1
22	28	29	20	15	-40.0	-25.0
29	30	23	33	27	145.5	-18.2
112	114	136	121	123	24.2	1.7

Table 4 (cont.)

State	1989	1990	1991	1992	1993	1994
New Mexico	26	21	34	33	33	40
New York	244	267	227	268	221	258
North Carolina	115	97	109	115	157	196
North Dakota	11	11	13	13	17	23
Ohio	158	198	178	186	187	199
Oklahoma	59	74	52	81	81	107
Oregon	50	45	55	67	63	41
Pennsylvania	153	155	176	179	187	186
Puerto Rico	24	35	43	48	37	47
Rhode Island	7	13	10	12	13	23
South Carolina	35	35	26	30	51	57
South Dakota	4	10	9	12	4	5
Tennessee	74	65	73	78	93	112
Texas	229	252	293	282	312	347
Utah	16	17	17	32	29	32
Vermont	17	13	5	11	16	16
Virginia	120	109	110	128	117	155
Virgin Islands	—	1	—	1	2	3
Washington	92	64	92	107	149	138
West Virginia	12	18	18	25	25	24
Wisconsin	104	96	126	130	134	172
Wyoming	9	11	14	15	16	19
UNITED STATES	3,890	3,916	4,247	4,651	4,767	5,373
Foreign	32	39	44	47	34	33
Missing	—	—	5	11	156	180
GRAND TOTAL	3,922	3,955	4,296	4,709	4,957	5,586

Due to multiple sources of data for each applicant, the total count per state may exceed the total number of applicants.

1995	1996	1997	1998	1999	*% Change 1989-99*	*% Change 1998-99*
45	40	45	42	49	88.5	16.7
404	282	308	276	306	25.4	10.9
223	192	201	203	243	111.3	19.7
38	70	24	28	13	18.2	-53.6
257	264	313	343	327	107.0	-4.7
123	128	132	126	118	100.0	-6.3
88	74	91	117	116	132.0	-0.9
247	210	227	228	270	76.5	18.4
53	50	65	60	46	91.7	-23.3
17	9	17	23	16	128.6	-30.4
44	57	66	66	64	82.9	-3.0
33	25	27	38	30	650.0	-21.1
117	126	152	143	160	116.2	11.9
396	394	408	427	405	76.9	-5.2
34	45	43	44	32	100.0	-27.3
11	9	12	15	16	-5.9	6.7
174	167	179	162	151	25.8	-6.8
1	4	2	—	2	—	—
143	171	193	175	163	77.2	-6.9
23	102	34	33	32	166.7	-3.0
178	186	148	166	176	69.2	6.0
23	15	18	33	25	177.8	-24.2
6,470	6,282	6,672	6,743	6,701	72.3	-0.6
50	16	14	54	10	-68.8	-81.5
81	203	81	76	70	—	-7.9
6,634	6,501	6,767	6,873	6,781	72.9	-1.3

Table 5
Number of Applications per Applicant by Residence, 1999

State	Applicants	Number of Applicants Submitting One or More Applications				
		1	2	3	4	5
Alabama	153	113	12	9	6	5
Alaska	7	2	0	0	0	0
Arizona	74	3	2	18	12	8
Arkansas	36	10	10	5	5	2
California	538	119	34	40	53	47
Colorado	350	282	7	7	11	10
Connecticut	50	7	3	3	4	2
Delaware	18	3	0	0	0	0
Dist. of Col.	1	1	0	0	0	0
Florida	265	58	31	42	30	19
Georgia	239	112	35	23	21	13
Hawaii	24	1	0	4	4	2
Idaho	41	22	6	7	0	4
Illinois	263	76	24	37	27	26
Indiana	126	55	16	15	11	9
Iowa	128	109	3	5	3	3
Kansas	118	99	8	2	2	2
Kentucky	102	69	8	5	8	2
Louisiana	202	165	12	10	5	3
Maine	11	4	2	1	1	1
Maryland	144	31	14	9	14	19
Massachusetts	182	81	2	14	12	10
Michigan	226	98	37	23	20	15
Minnesota	137	71	21	25	8	3
Mississippi	79	67	2	1	2	1
Missouri	158	142	4	1	3	4
Montana	39	3	7	12	10	1
Nebraska	65	48	6	3	3	3
Nevada	15	2	1	0	2	3
New Hampshire	27	8	0	3	1	1

6	7	8	9	10	>10	Total Applications	Applications per Applicants
4	2	0	1	1	0	270	1.76
0	3	1	1	0	0	40	5.71
5	3	4	3	2	14	482	6.51
1	0	1	0	0	2	112	3.11
34	38	25	21	21	106	3,424	6.36
8	10	5	3	1	6	690	1.97
8	3	1	2	5	12	377	7.54
2	5	1	3	0	4	145	8.06
0	0	0	0	0	0	1	1.00
23	11	9	7	11	24	1,274	4.81
8	9	4	4	2	8	722	3.02
4	3	1	1	1	3	153	6.38
0	1	0	0	0	1	96	2.34
24	17	5	13	5	9	1,087	4.13
6	6	0	3	0	5	404	3.21
1	1	2	1	0	0	195	1.52
4	0	0	0	0	1	174	1.47
4	2	3	0	0	1	219	2.15
2	2	2	0	0	1	309	1.53
0	1	1	0	0	0	35	3.18
11	21	5	6	2	12	744	5.17
9	6	9	3	8	28	869	4.77
12	11	0	3	2	5	653	2.89
4	0	1	0	1	3	314	2.29
3	1	0	0	1	1	133	1.68
3	1	0	0	0	0	210	1.33
3	2	0	0	0	1	150	3.85
0	1	0	0	1	0	113	1.74
0	1	4	1	0	1	86	5.73
3	4	1	2	1	3	148	5.48

Table 5 (cont.)

State	Applicants	Number of Applicants Submitting One or More Applications				
		1	*2*	*3*	*4*	*5*
New Jersey	123	18	7	9	5	11
New Mexico	49	14	3	10	5	3
New York	306	45	24	27	33	25
North Carolina	243	133	24	18	25	13
North Dakota	13	2	1	2	2	3
Ohio	327	241	14	18	11	11
Oklahoma	118	82	8	10	6	4
Oregon	116	59	23	7	7	13
Pennsylvania	270	54	21	25	37	29
Puerto Rico	46	13	4	6	4	2
Rhode Island	16	9	1	0	1	1
South Carolina	64	23	7	8	7	8
South Dakota	30	15	6	4	3	1
Tennessee	160	104	16	12	8	9
Texas	405	214	68	42	26	15
Utah	32	3	0	8	2	2
Vermont	16	4	2	1	1	0
Virginia	151	55	21	17	15	10
Virgin Islands	2	0	0	0	0	1
Washington	163	76	18	22	8	9
West Virginia	32	6	8	6	4	3
Wisconsin	176	81	34	23	10	7
Wyoming	25	7	1	2	4	6
UNITED STATES	6,701	3,119	618	601	502	404
Foreign	10	8	0	0	0	0
Unknown	70	29	9	9	7	2
GRAND TOTAL	6,781	3,156	627	610	509	406

Due to multiple sources of data for each applicant, the total count per state may exceed the total number of applicants.

6	7	8	9	10	>10	Total Applications	Applications per Applicant
8	8	9	5	11	32	973	7.91
1	4	2	4	0	3	209	4.27
25	26	18	15	14	54	2,005	6.55
11	5	5	0	1	8	668	2.75
1	1	0	0	0	1	62	4.77
10	8	4	5	0	5	690	2.11
1	4	0	2	0	1	247	2.09
2	1	1	1	0	2	282	2.43
32	16	14	11	9	22	1,412	5.23
3	4	1	2	2	5	230	5.00
2	0	0	0	0	2	58	3.63
2	2	5	0	0	2	219	3.42
1	0	0	0	0	0	62	2.07
3	2	3	0	1	2	344	2.15
8	9	2	4	2	15	1,049	2.59
5	5	1	1	1	4	190	5.94
1	2	2	0	1	2	95	5.94
5	9	2	6	1	10	564	3.74
0	1	0	0	0	0	12	6.00
7	6	11	1	2	3	498	3.06
3	1	0	1	0	0	105	3.28
3	7	3	1	2	5	475	2.70
2	1	0	1	0	1	100	4.00
322	287	168	138	112	430	24,178	3.61
0	0	2	0	0	0	24	2.40
1	1	3	0	6	3	246	3.51
323	288	173	138	118	433	24,448	3.61

Table 6

Applicants to U.S. Colleges of Veterinary Medicine by Ethnicity and Gender, 1987-1999

	Year	Total Applicants	Caucasian	Minority* Applicants	African-American
Total	1987	4,758	4,106	326	104
Applicants	1988	4,509	3,891	309	110
	1989	3,922	3,619	303	90
	1990	3,955	3,639	316	88
	1991	4,296	3,900	356	100
	1992	4,709	4,210	402	109
	1993	4,957	4,300	579	115
	1994	5,428	4,775	603	132
	1995	6,634	5,966	567	138
	1996	6,424	5,426	721	110
	1997	6,630	5,726	704	132
	1998	6,783	5,720	745	149
	1999	6,695	5,648	708	135
Male	1987	2,019	1,717	151	49
Applicants	1988	1,827	1,551	138	48
	1989	1,490	1,367	123	30
	1990	1,465	1,344	121	24
	1991	1,507	1,349	149	44
	1992	1,613	1,431	148	36
	1993	1,719	1,484	208	37
	1994	1,810	1,575	212	43
	1995	2,158	1,931	195	40
	1996	2,027	1,703	227	31
	1997	2,005	1,739	201	33
	1998	2,015	1,689	225	43
	1999	1,846	1,539	198	37
Female	1987	2,739	2,389	175	55
Applicants	1988	2,682	2,340	171	62
	1989	2,432	2,252	180	60
	1990	2,490	2,295	195	64
	1991	2,789	2,551	207	56
	1992	3,096	2,779	254	73
	1993	3,238	2,816	371	78
	1994	3,618	3,200	391	89
	1995	4,476	4,035	372	98
	1996	4,397	3,723	494	79
	1997	4,625	3,987	503	99
	1998	4,768	4,031	520	106
	1999	4,849	4,109	510	98

* Minority totals exclude unknown/unreported ethnic identity numbers.

Hispanic	Native Amer/ Alaskan	Asian/Polynesian	Other	Unreported/ Unknown
141	25	56		
117	23	59		
121	23	69		
122	22	84		
148	22	86		40
176	43	74		97
180	45	239		78
184	58	229		50
200	42	154	33	101
233	59	277	42	277
242	67	189	74	200
243	75	206	72	318
226	55	204	88	339
69	12	21		
58	12	20		
58	11	24		
61	9	27		
67	11	27		9
77	13	22		34
69	13	89		27
79	21	69		23
70	14	54	17	32
78	20	85	13	97
72	23	48	25	65
77	29	50	26	101
71	17	50	23	109
72	13	35		
59	11	39		
63	12	45		
61	13	57		
81	11	59		31
99	30	52		63
111	32	150		51
105	37	160		27
130	28	100	16	69
155	39	192	29	180
170	44	141	49	135
166	46	156	46	217
155	38	154	65	230

Table 7

Acceptances by Gender, 1995-99

	1995			1996		
	Applications	Acceptances	Percent Accepted	Applications	Acceptances	Percent Accepted
MALE	2,158	741	34.3	2,027	779	38.4
New Applicants	1,564	544	34.8	1,480	584	39.5
Repeat Applicants	594	197	33.2	548	195	35.6
FEMALE	4,476	1,539	34.4	4.397	1,514	34.4
New Applicants	3,315	1,170	35.3	3,260	1,156	35.5
Repeat Applicants	1,161	369	31.8	1,137	358	31.5
TOTAL	6,634	2,280	34.4	6,424	2,293	35.7
New Applicants	4,879	1,714	35.1	4,740	1,740	36.7
Repeat Applicants	1,755	566	32.3	1,685	553	32.8

Applications, Applicants, and Positions, U.S. Colleges of Veterinary Medicine, 1980-99

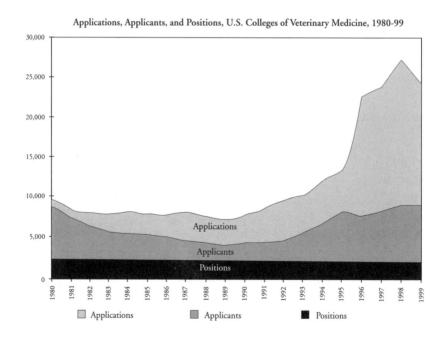

Applications, Applicants, and Positions, U.S. Colleges of Veterinary Medicine, 1980-99

1997			1998			1999*		
Applications	Acceptances	Percent Accepted	Applications	Acceptances	Percent Accepted	Applications	Acceptances	Percent Accepted
2,005	665	33.17	2,015	617	30.62	1,846	622	33.69
1,415	488	34.49	1,319	424	32.15	1,172	414	35.32
590	177	30.00	696	193	27.73	674	208	30.86
4,625	1,542	33.34	4,768	1,572	32.97	4,849	1,576	32.50
3,285	1,166	35.49	3,158	1,104	34.96	3,157	1,107	35.06
1,340	376	28.06	1,610	468	29.07	1,692	469	27.72
6,630	2,207	33.29	6,783	2,189	32.27	6,695	2,198	32.83
4,700	1,654	35.19	4,477	1,528	34.13	4,329	1,521	35.14
1,930	553	28.65	2,306	661	28.66	2,366	677	28.61

* Does not represent final acceptance numbers

New and Repeat Applicants, U.S. Colleges of Veterinary Medicine, 1984-1999

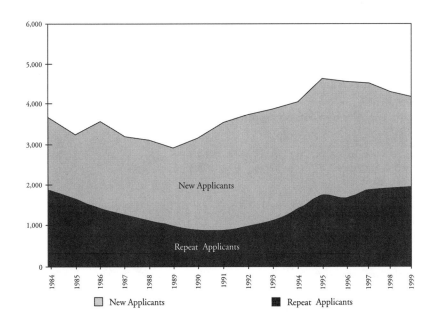

163

Table 8

Ethnic Identity of VMCAS Applicants by Institution, 1999

School	African American	Hispanic American	Mexican American	Other Latino	American Indian	Filipino American	Chinese American
Auburn	8	18	2	9	5	2	7
UCDavis	15	23	22	19	12	4	43
Cornell	25	33	14	15	7	3	29
Florida	22	32	3	14	5	0	13
Georgia	15	19	3	9	6	4	8
Illinois	16	20	8	12	6	4	23
Iowa	11	23	2	11	8	3	16
Kansas	4	20	3	8	6	2	8
Louisiana	22	44	11	20	11	3	15
Michigan	24	32	14	17	12	4	23
Minnesota	20	21	13	12	9	5	18
Mississippi	3	11	5	8	5	3	4
N Carolina	27	29	8	19	6	3	13
Ohio	9	16	2	13	3	1	15
Oklahoma	1	14	5	7	19	1	3
Oregon	10	26	12	12	11	2	22
UPenn	23	26	13	15	4	4	30
Purdue	19	16	9	17	4	1	16
Tennessee	16	9	2	4	6	1	3
Texas A&M	12	28	12	15	8	2	16
VA-MD Reg.	20	16	4	8	4	3	17
Washington	10	24	13	14	13	4	25
Wisconsin	13	30	14	13	8	4	24
U.S. Subtotal	345	530	194	291	178	63	391
UPEI	8	14	5	6	4	1	10
Guelph	0	0	0	2	0	0	0
TOTAL	353	544	199	299	182	64	401

Table 9

Ethnic Identity of VMCAS Applicants, 1999

Ethnic Identity	Males	Females	Unknown	Total
African American	19	64	0	83
Hispanic American	36	73	0	109
Mexican American	11	35	0	46
Other Latino	13	27	0	40
American Indian	14	32	0	46
Filipino American	3	10	0	13
Chinese American	11	50	0	61
East Indian	5	8	0	13
Japanese American	8	28	0	36
Korean American	10	25	0	35
Pacific Islander	2	2	0	4
Other Asian	7	16	0	23
White	1,138	3,168	0	4,306
Other	15	45	1	61
Declined to state	102	259	37	398
TOTAL	1,394	3,842	38	5,274

East Indian	Japanese American	Korean American	Pacific Islander	Other Asian	White	Other	Declined to State	Total
1	3	5	1	2	505	3	42	613
6	23	17	3	8	731	20	112	1,058
6	6	13	0	6	944	20	118	1,239
2	6	5	2	7	632	13	56	812
1	2	5	0	4	670	12	62	820
7	6	12	0	5	835	12	107	1,073
5	6	6	1	1	797	10	67	967
2	5	4	0	0	421	8	38	529
1	9	7	1	5	907	15	73	1,144
6	13	14	0	6	1,033	16	103	1,317
3	9	8	1	4	824	13	76	1,036
1	3	3	0	0	315	2	32	395
3	9	13	1	7	916	12	84	1,150
1	8	7	0	3	555	6	59	698
1	3	3	1	0	375	6	31	470
1	19	10	1	4	752	17	87	986
9	13	16	0	7	1,055	20	143	1,378
7	8	6	1	4	748	18	73	947
1	3	1	0	2	377	7	31	463
2	8	4	2	8	773	7	58	955
4	4	8	0	5	800	6	93	992
2	21	12	2	6	828	16	100	1,090
8	8	8	1	6	1,051	17	121	1,326
80	195	187	18	100	16,844	276	1,766	21,458
1	1	5	1	1	307	10	44	418
1	0	0	0	0	20	1	5	29
82	196	192	19	101	17,171	287	1,815	21,905

Table 10
VMCAS Offers of Admission by Ethnic Identity, 1999

Ethnic Identity	Male	Female	Unknown	Total
African American	7	25	0	32
Hispanic American	12	18	0	30
Mexican American	2	17	0	19
Other Latino	3	12	0	15
American Indian	2	10	0	12
Filipino American	0	0	0	0
Chinese American	10	40	0	50
East Indian	4	6	0	10
Japanese American	1	23	0	24
Korean American	0	9	0	9
Pacific Islander	0	0	0	0
Other Asian	5	7	0	12
White	483	1,345	0	1,828
Other	0	10	0	10
Declined to state	50	101	19	170
TOTAL	579	1,623	19	2,221

Table 11
Historical Summary of VMCAS Applications and Applicants, 1996–1999

	1995–96	1996–97	1997–98	1998–99
Full Participating Schools	14	13	18	18
Partial Participating (Required for Non-Residents)	4	6	3	3
Partial Participating (Optional for Non-Residents)	4	4	3	4
VMCAS Applications (complete)	18,493	19,217	24,766	21,905
VMCAS Applicants (complete)	4,378	4,378	5,350	5,274
Percent Accepted	28.43	29.78	31.03	31.73
Applications per Applicant Ratio	4.2	4.4	4.6	4.1
REPEAT* VMCAS Applicants	0	994	1,308	1,515
NEW VMCAS Applicants	4,378	3,384	4,042	3,759

* "Repeat VMCAS Applicants" indicates only those applicants who have applied through the service in a previous cycle.

Table 12
Number of VMCAS Applications per Applicant, 1999–2000

		Offers per Applicant							
Applications	Applicants	0	1	2	3	4	5	6	>6
1	1,760	1,202	558	0	0	0	0	0	0
2	670	468	174	28	0	0	0	0	0
3	603	422	152	23	6	0	0	0	0
4	479	326	115	30	8	0	0	0	0
5	401	267	90	30	9	4	1	0	0
6	320	208	78	17	8	8	1	0	0
7	233	152	48	27	6	0	0	0	0
8	162	101	32	15	9	4	0	1	0
9	131	87	21	16	1	1	4	1	0
10	129	93	18	10	2	3	2	1	0
11	69	48	10	9	2	0	0	0	0
12	58	43	7	3	2	2	1	0	0
13	52	37	6	5	2	1	1	0	0
14	40	30	4	3	2	1	0	0	0
15	35	20	7	1	3	3	0	1	0
16	25	12	7	1	2	2	0	1	0
17	17	12	2	0	0	2	0	1	0
18	19	14	5	0	0	0	0	0	0
19	14	10	2	2	0	0	0	0	0
20	11	4	2	2	1	1	0	0	1
21	13	11	1	1	0	0	0	0	0
22	12	5	3	3	0	0	0	1	0
23	9	6	2	0	0	0	0	1	0
24	10	8	2	0	0	0	0	0	0
25	2	1	1	0	0	0	0	0	0
Total	5,274	3,587	1,347	226	63	32	10	8	1

St. Louis Community College
at Meramec
Library